THE
HOSPITAL
THAT
ATE
CHICAGO

For Bob Aber —

With the very warmest
feeling and high respect —

Sege Lahm

1978 TOTAL NATIONAL HEALTH CARE EXPENDITURES
$192.4 Billion = 9.1% GNP

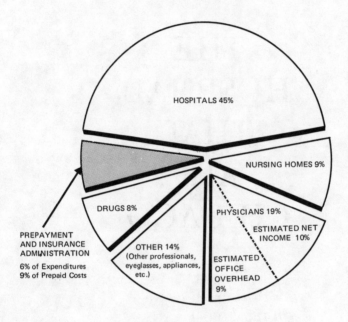

HOSPITALS 45%

NURSING HOMES 9%

DRUGS 8%

PHYSICIANS 19%

ESTIMATED NET INCOME 10%

PREPAYMENT AND INSURANCE ADMINISTRATION

6% of Expenditures
9% of Prepaid Costs

OTHER 14%
(Other professionals, eyeglasses, appliances, etc.)

ESTIMATED OFFICE OVERHEAD 9%

PLUS: RESEARCH $4.3 Billion and PUBLIC HEALTH ACTIVITY ($5.1 Billion) = $192.4 Billion

SOURCE: HCFA SURVEY, Summer 1979

THE HOSPITAL THAT ATE CHICAGO

Distortions Imposed on the Medical System by Its Financing

George Ross Fisher, M.D.

THE SAUNDERS PRESS
W. B. Saunders Company
Philadelphia • London • Toronto

The Saunders Press
W. B. Saunders Company
West Washington Square
Philadelphia, PA 19105

IN THE UNITED STATES DISTRIBUTED TO THE TRADE BY
HOLT, RINEHART & WINSTON
383 Madison Avenue
New York, NY 10017

IN CANADA DISTRIBUTED BY
HOLT, RINEHART & WINSTON OF CANADA, LTD.
55 Horner Avenue
Toronto, Ontario
M8Z 4X6
Canada

Grateful acknowledgement is made to the *New England Journal of Medicine* for permission
to reprint "The Hospital That Ate Chicago." (Volume #301 Number 1; July 5, 1979)

Library of Congress Cataloging in Publication Data

Fisher, George Ross.
  The hospital that ate Chicago.

  1. Medical care, Cost of—United States.
2. Hospitals—United States—Cost of operation.
3. Medical economics—United States.   4. Health
maintenance organizations—United States—Finance.
I. Title.
RA410.53.F57   338.4'3362110973   79-76113
ISBN 0-7216-3707-8

Library of Congress Catalog Card Number: 79-67114

W. B. Saunders Company ISBN NO: 0-7216-3707-8
Holt, Rinehart & Winston ISBN NO: 0-03-056741-6

Print Number 9 8 7 6 5 4 3 2
                                    First Edition

Printed in the United States of America

Contents

Introduction

This book was written to stimulate public awareness of a problem which, apparently, only the public can resolve. I have spent considerable time and effort in past years working through the normal channels on what superficially appear to be obscure technical problems of insurance, finance, and hospital organization. The principal conclusion which came to me was that all of those affected by the problem are trapped by the overlapping constraints of a system which, though it has evolved from good motives, was based on two inappropriate premises.

The first premise was that modern health care is such a fundamental right of all citizens that it ought to be subsidized by income tax concessions. The second premise is that the insurance mechanism is an appropriate way to finance the entire health system.

The distortions in the present complicated health finance tangle grow out of the logical, meticulous, and energetic elaboration of these two basic premises. In the burlesques, sketches, and fictional asides which are scattered through the present serious discussion, the name O'Toole is used to symbolize those honorable and well-meaning people who have made the situation worse by logical expansion of the premises which I believe to be faulty. Nothing ethnic or personal is intended by this name, and to all those whose real name is O'Toole, I apologize.

A great many people helped me with the material for this book, and I have used some of their names in the fictional episodes. They have been asked, and they don't mind. Naturally, there are other people who have the same name, and some of them may work in similar fields or have had similar experiences. To them I must also apologize, and hope they will understand that a fictional character has to have a name which has a normal sound to it.

There are two rather complicated obscurities which must become part of common American parlance if the American public is to understand how medical care is being distorted by its financing arrangement. One is termed "contractual allowance," and the other is "retrospective cost reimbursement." Don't run away. You must try to understand at least the outline of these mysteries if you are to permit your elected representatives and your community leaders to face possible unpopularity when they try to change them. This book has attempted to make these issues clear by any trick of illustration which my imagination could devise. I suppose I will be accused of oversimplifying, but in trying these ideas out on my friends I became convinced that these issues are impervious to oversimplification.

If the reader already happens to understand the issues, he can jump to the set of solutions I propose in the second half of the book. No doubt some will find the proposed solutions so distasteful that they will then return to the first half of the book to search out where I went wrong. Fine. Now we can have a discussion.

It happens that I am not one of the critics of our system who despair of the political process. In my experience, politicians have a special talent for simplifying complicated issues into one-liners, carefully exploring the power and motives of provoked resistance, and devising workable compromises toward the best achievable result. Politicans should be allowed to work these things out their way, which is a good way. But they cannot work efficiently with a vital issue like health care if they are blocked by universal public ignorance of what is at stake.

A number of earnest people are probably going to think they are under attack in this book. They aren't, and I'm sorry if they feel that they are. I can only console myself that I tried not to stack the deck, and that to be ignored would be worse than being misquoted. If such people find that I have made errors, which I probably have, I hope they will stop to ask whether the errors really affect the substance of the argument. The issue is not my credibility, it is the credibility of the argument.

Finally, let me extend my particular thanks to James Rahn who gave me many insights into hospital accounting. And to my family "editorial board" for their help. Especially thanks to my son, George, who suggested the title, and Howard E. Sandum, my editor, who encouraged me to make it the theme of the book.

G.R.F.
Philadelphia, September 11, 1979

1

The Hospital that Ate Chicago

Once upon a time, there was a hospital accountant named Stephen Girard O'Toole. His father had been one of the poor white orphan boys educated at Girard College, hence the son's name. As with most accountants, young Stephen grew up deeply impressed with the power of tax-free compound interest, particularly when harnessed with a shrewdly written last will and testament. He was drawn to hospital work when he discovered that his initials (S.G.O.T.) carried scientific significance.

For some years before our story begins, Mr. O'Toole (as he came to be styled) had been using his talents, whenever the opportunity appeared, to promote flower bonds. A flower bond is a United States Treasury bond, with a kicker. Such bonds can be purchased at considerably less than face value, but are worth full face value for the payment of federal estate taxes. Since they can be bought by making a telephone call as little as an hour before the owner dies, they are a last chance for any wealthy person on the brink, so to speak. It was therefore Mr. O'Toole's practice to suggest flower bonds to certain patients in the more expensive private rooms of his hospital. The Medical Records department reported to the financial division of the hospital, so Mr. O'Toole had little trouble checking on a diagnosis. This saved him the embarrassment of proposing flower bonds to mere hypochondriacs.

One day, Mr. O'Toole was making flower bond rounds when he encountered a dear old dying lady named Mrs. O'Leary. Mrs. O'Leary was delighted to be visited by anybody, since she had no living relatives. Accordingly, although she had no particular interest in reducing her estate taxes, she saw that Mr. O'Toole wanted to talk about bonds, so bonds it was. In keeping with a time-honored custom of her sex, she talked about what *she* wanted to talk about, which was slum clearance, urban renewal, and the elimination of unemployment. Now and then, flower bonds were mentioned in order to entice Mr. O'Toole into coming back the next day.

Their pleasant conversational games went on for several days before a grand new thought struck Mr. O'Toole. Here was the perfect prospect for a will that would out-Girard Stephen Girard! That evening he opened the subject.

"Mrs. O'Leary, have you taken the precaution to write a will?"

The old lady smiled sweetly. "Yes, of course, I've left my whole estate to Ralph Nader, for slum clearance and the elimination of unemployment."

"And you've given thought to minimizing estate taxes?"

"Well, dear boy, the government can use the tax money to clear slums and reduce unemployment, too. Ralph Nader will see that they do."

Mr. O'Toole suppressed his own opinion of Ralph Nader. Slums and unemployment, however, would serve the purpose at hand. "I wonder," he said, "if you have ever considered the effect of building hospitals on the clearing of slums and the alleviation of unemployment?"

Mrs. O'Leary expressed surprise that the clearing of a few downtown blocks could have any impact like that of a dynamic organization devoted to molding public opinion and shaping government policy. There was suddenly a glint in O'Toole's eyes.

"If you will patiently listen, I will show you how a single hospital could clean up Philadelphia in fifty years."

"Chicago," she replied.

"I beg your pardon?" asked a startled O'Toole.

"My grandfather made his money in the Chicago dairy business. If we are to talk of cleaning up any city, it is going to be Chicago."

Since it was obvious that the choice of cities was a closed issue, O'Toole shrugged his shoulders and pressed on with the proposal.

"You may not realize it, dear lady, but substantially all the income of a hospital comes from third-party—ah, excuse me, *insurance* payments. They pay us our costs. And one of our costs is the reality that the building is gradually wearing out. Another cost is the interest we must pay on our mortgage."

Mrs. O'Leary had grown up in a world of small investments, and was not nearly as dotty as she acted. "You mean," she asked, "that a hospital doesn't care if interest rates are high?"

"I mean," answered O'Toole, "that a nonprofit hospital likes interest rates to be as high as possible. When the hospital borrows money, the interest is reimbursed. On the other hand, when it invests money, the interest is tax-exempt. You will see that this is an important point in what I have to propose to you."

"I'm way ahead of you, young man. You are suggesting that a hospital can invest money which it obtained through what amounts to an interest-free loan. And tax-exempt, no less. Put compound interest to work on that, and in fifty years you would own the earth, young man."

Mr. O'Toole saw that he had hooked his fish. He asked her to think about the subject overnight; he would return the following evening with more details, and when he did, Mrs. O'Leary had a list of written questions.

"First of all, what do you need my money for?" she asked. "Why doesn't the hospital go ahead and borrow the bank dry?"

"Well," said O'Toole, "you can't be reimbursed by insurance companies for just any loan. It has to be related to some patient care purpose, like a mortgage or accounts receivable—oh, pardon me, *unpaid bills.*"

"Is that why you didn't send me a bill for three months after my last hospitalization?"

At this, O'Toole colored slightly. This old girl may have been dying but she wasn't dead by a long shot.

"Now, let's examine a little problem we have in cash shortage whenever we build a building," O'Toole said moving briskly along into safer territory. "The hospital gets paid for the building wearing out over forty years. But the bank wants its mortgage paid off in twenty years. We have it made after twenty years, but we need to prime the pump."

Mrs. O'Leary considered the matter briefly. "Are you suggesting that I should put up half the cost of a new building? I'm comfortable, but I don't have that kind of money. These hospitals cost $100 million, nowadays."

"Well," said the financial man, "with the right kind of arrangement, the thing can be arranged for between 5 percent and 10 percent of the building cost as up-front money. The money isn't consumed, by the way. When it eventually returns, the process starts over again."

Mrs. O'Leary pondered the matter; it was true she could afford that. However, she knew that the best way to get rid of Mr. O'Toole would be to tell him she didn't have the money. She had to hold back until she decided whether or not he was going to be a pest.

Mr. O'Toole, on the other hand, could not know what she was thinking. Her silence might mean indecision, and he wished to keep the subject alive with more details.

"Let me tell you about these mortgages. Only a small part of the early payments go to retire the principal of the loan, the rest is interest. Since I've explained that the loan is essentially interest-free, the important thing is that the repayment of principal in the early years is small. Smaller than the depreciation—ah, excuse me, smaller than the amount the insurance companies pay us for the gradual wearing out of the building. So, in the first five years we make a profit, which we invest. The investment pays for the second five years. We only need your money for the second ten years; if you give it to us now, we can invest it and double it by the time we need it."

"You can do better than that with the money, young fellow," she began in a menacing way, and he instantly agreed. One high roller knew how to talk to another. It was the principle that mattered.

"Now let me go on," said the young man. "Perhaps you can see how these things overlap. The extra cash you generate in a new building helps to pay the cash shortage on the building which is ten years old. And the extra depreciation payments on a building twenty years old make up any difference. Take my word for it, the best way to arrange the finance of a hospital is to build it in a series of seven pavilions, one every five years."

"Well," said Mrs. O'Leary, "I'm sure that's all very clever and important. But I don't really see it as a way to clear slums, whereas Mr. Nader . . ."

"Please forgive me for interrupting," said O'Toole, "but there is a point I haven't mentioned. You will notice that the seven-pavilion system assumes that you will tear down the oldest pavilion in order to make room for the new one. But a forty-year-old hospital is still a useful building, even if it is all paid up.

"My proposal is that we just let it stand, and keep on building pavilions at a rate that will accelerate as the depreciation starts rolling in. I calculate that you could convert all the slums of Chicago into hospital pavilions in another fifty years after you got rolling."

Mrs. O'Leary pondered, then asked, "But where would all those people live?"

"Very simple. They would become hospital employees. That solves the unemployment problem too. You may wonder whether there would be enough patients to fill all the beds, but that can be accomplished by increasing the ratio of employees to patients. At the present time the average is four employees per patient, but it is growing fast. There are already two local hospitals with a ratio of 7.5 to one; and it only needs to reach 100 to one to take care of the patient shortage."

"Whatever the ratio is in this hospital right now," the lady tartly remarked, "it isn't enough to get someone to answer the buzzer."

"You see what I mean," grinned O'Toole.

"Yes, I do. Call my lawyer, young man. I'm going to write a will."

2

Why Do Hospitals Cost So Much?

Like most doctors, I know almost nothing about the construction finances and cost accounting policies of the hospitals where I am associated. Indeed, I could not even tell you the names or the office locations of their cost accountants. Whatever this book may be, it is not an oblique attack on any particular hospital, especially those particular hospitals. It is not an exposé of what their accountants have told me. The hospital that ate Chicago exists only as an imaginary device, a fable. Its purpose is to stimulate curiosity about a subject which is moderately difficult to understand, but which can be understood by any reader willing to try. There will be other burlesques and fables scattered through the book, which are meant to illustrate, to puzzle, to explain, and to encourage the reader to make just a little effort to understand how hospitals and all other parts of the health system are twisting in a net of insurance.

That's really what this book is about: Insurance. But we must first spend a long while on the much more interesting subject of hospitals. As we see how the financing system torments these institutions into behavior which sometimes is imperfect, the intrinsically dull subject of insurance begins to take on a fascination. If you are interested in hospitals, you will soon be interested in health insurance and you might grow impassioned about it. We begin with the financial characteristic of hospitals which most people think they understand very clearly. Hospitals cost a lot.

The chilling thing, however, about the title of this chapter is that it may sound out-dated. "Why do hospitals cost so much?" was a lively question fifteen years ago, but now the public has almost stopped asking it. People seem to think they might as well have

FIGURE 1

Increases in the Consumer Price Index and the Hospital Room Charge and Medical Care Components 1974 - 1978

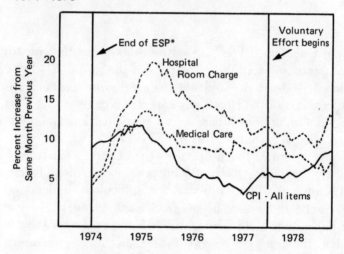

Source: U.S. Bureau of Labor Statistics, CPI through 1977, CPI-W in 1978.

*Economic Stabilization Program

NOTE: Definition of Hospital Room Charge component was changed in January 1978 from semi-private rooms to include all types of accommodations including private and intensive care rooms. The hospital components of the CPI overstate inflation in the industry for two reasons. First, the hospital components of the CPI are not weighted averages of all hospital products because the prices sampled apply only to those purchasers paying full charges. Second, in addition to unit price change, the hospital components pick up the effects of increases in quantity and service intensity on unit price, which also results in an overstatement of the rate of inflation.

asked why aircraft carriers cost so much, for all the enlightenment that emerged, or for all the difference it made. Hospitals and aircraft carriers are expensive, that's all. The public now only asks whether we need so many of them, and how to arrange to pay for the ones we have. Among doctors, however, the basic cost question continues to be asked uneasily, in the spirit the public used to ask it. The prices really don't seem appropriate for what you get.

One simplistic line of reasoning goes as follows. A man and his wife apparently can check into a first-class hotel, order all meals from room service, and hire round-the-clock nurses for less than it costs to be in a hospital. Their itemized daily bill might be:

Twin-Bed Room for Two	$ 60
Room Service Meals for Two	45
Three Shifts of Private Nurses	195
Total	$300
	($150 per person per day)[1]

You could find cheaper hotels, but let's not stack the deck. Hotels make no bones about seeking a profit, and a private nurse for two people provides considerably more nursing intensity than is necessary or customary in contemporary acute-care hospitals. Hospital food costs per patient day are less than a hotel would charge, perhaps only half as much.

In a hospital as in a hotel, housekeeping, billing, room reservation, security, and telephone support services must be provided. In an acute-care hospital, a floor of forty patients may share the services of a twenty-member nursing team, paid at a lower average rate than private-duty graduate nurses are paid. Twenty nurses for forty patients may sound the same as one private-duty for two people; that isn't so, because the team has to work three shifts and cover weekends. Each hospital patient gets the equivalent in services of about one-third of a full-time nurse each day. Perhaps some hospitals provide as much as one-half, full-time equivalent (FTE) per patient day. Now, let's add up the daily hospital bill on the same conjectural basis as we did for the hotel room:

1. It could be argued that we should include $23 for daily service by a resident physician. However, this is one of the indirect costs we will be discussing later. Not every hospital provides residents, and when they do the cost is often disproportionately included in the charges for intensive care units.

Semiprivate Room for Two	$ 60
Meals for Two	25
Nursing Service for Two	70
(at ½ FTE[2] per patient Day)	$155
	($77.50 per patient per day)

It becomes clear from even such a rough outline that a hospital actually does produce some economies by concentrating patients in one place, feeding them minimal-choice dormitory food, and employing lesser-skilled (i.e., lesser-paid) employees to concentrate the use of registered nurses to functions for which RN's alone have training. Economies of scale. It would look as though a forty-bed hospital would be about half as expensive as do-it-yourself care in a hotel. Half as expensive, perhaps, but the cost savings do not seem to reach the patient. Some other internal profit eats up the economies of scale for its own purposes. After all, most hospitals are now charging over two hundred dollars a day. The average hospital has, not merely one-half nurse per patient, but three full-time equivalent employees of all sorts per patient. Who are they, and do we need them?

Now, let's not get excited. A hospital provides a great many services which are not obtainable in a hotel. If those services are broken out and charged for separately, then of course they cannot be counted as part of the daily cost of running the institution; in this sense, the operating rooms, laboratories, and X-ray departments do not count. By analogy, it is handy to have a drug store in the lobby of the hotel, but you do not pay extra on your hotel bill for this convenience; the drug store makes its own charges, just as the operating room does. It would seem some other services must be provided to the patients in a hospital which are not separately charged for, but which effectively double the price of the room.

These would be called unitemized, indirect, overhead costs. We are not going to pause at this point to list or describe the indirect costs, since it will take much of the rest of the book to make the matter comprehensible. But perhaps the beacon can be lit. The basic daily cost of a hospital is nearly doubled by the existence of

2. Full-time equivalent, mixing graduate nurses, practical nurses, aides, orderlies, and clerks. The salary is estimated on the high side, to minimize quibbling.

indirect costs which are invisible to the patients and even baffling to the doctors.

The title of this book, and the fictional burlesque which is the first chapter, light a second lantern for the reader. We are going to find that the construction of new hospital buildings plays a heavy role in the indirect cost of a hospital.

It will probably take a few chapters before the average reader can completely understand the joke about "the hospital that ate Chicago" which was dropped on him in the first chapter. But it is no accident that the joke is also the title of this book. The present rush of hospital construction is an absolutely central feature of the real mess we are in, because it constitutes the profit in the system, and profit drives every system to some degree. Let's give a preliminary hint. A nonprofit corporation may not make a profit. But a nonprofit corporation may definitely own a building.

Understanding this tangle is a process which needs careful instruction, and probably also requires spectacular illustration. Since, however, it is my conclusion that short-cut "solutions" of the facility construction issue would bring on still worse disasters, it must be confessed that the argument is held back from the reader until he has paid his dues by listening to a rehearsal of the underlying causes of the problem, and the larger implications of changing it. If someone is hopelessly in love with regulation, there is probably little hope of changing that person's mind. But nevertheless, no one is going to get tips for new regulations from this book until he has brushed his way past some proposals for eliminating regulation through strengthening the medical market-place. Strengthening the medical marketplace is clearly the remedy, but it is not an easy way out. By contrast, regulation is merely a temporary escape from facing the hard issues.

We will take up the issue of regulation versus strengthening market mechanisms in later chapters. The present question is why hospitals cost what they do. We have first taken a simple outsider's look at the daily nonprofit room-and-board charge, compared it with the going prices for profitable first-class hotels, and concluded that somewhere there must be some obscure indirect hospital costs which come close to doubling the price. Let's search for another comparison in order to make other conjectures which may turn out to be reassuring, or maybe turn out to be as disquieting as the hotel comparison. When the man was asked how his wife was, the old joke has him reply: "Compared with what?"

Since rising hospital costs have given concern for their inflationary effect on the national economy, useful insights can perhaps be gained from looking at hospital costs as a portion of the total national budget. Economists have given us a concept they call the gross national product (GNP) which is an estimate they somehow make of the total cost of everything the whole nation pays for in a year. Our gross national product is now roughly two trillion dollars. The cost of medical care, including everything from linaments to brain surgery to typing up Medicare invoices, is estimated to be rapidly growing from 8 to 10 percent of the GNP, which is itself also growing. Since all of this is only estimated anyway, it would not be too far wrong to place our annual national medical bill at $200 billion. That's pretty close to what we spend on national defense in peace time, and the nonprofit nature of most hospitals reduces income tax recapture, so health is really a little costlier and a little more inflationary than it looks. By placing 40 percent of hospital costs in the public sector, a second special inflationary mischief has been created by rising medical costs. Only the federal government can print money, and the federal health insurance programs cause the government to print plenty of it. To the extent that most of the Medicare and Medicaid payments go to nonprofit institutions, and thus escape taxation on the first pass, the inflationary impact when the money is passed out to employees and vendors is greater than similar expenditures for, say, national defense. If you didn't get that, let's say it again. You have more income to spend if you don't pay taxes.

So the 4 percent of gross national product (80 billion dollars) which each year flows to hospitals then flows on to others, in an after-tax proportion greater than is true of the defense industry. While inflationary effects are exaggerated by the nonprofit phenomenon, they are reduced by another internal characteristic. Recent trends toward hospital-centered medical care have caused a certain amount of cost shifting which appears to be, but actually is not, an escalation of hospital-induced expenditures. The hospital has become the purchasing agent for some things which were formerly considered nonhospital expenses. X-rays, for example, are now mostly taken in hospital X-ray departments, but until recent years there was a large and flourishing profession of office radiology.

Indeed, things have got to the point where states are being urged to pass laws forbidding the purchase of advanced X-ray equipment (the CAT or "Computerized Axial Tomography" Scanner) by radiologists for their offices, as if private ownership of X-ray equipment was some sort of underhanded trick. The radiologists themselves, like the pathologists and anaesthesiologists, may move from private practice to salaried arrangements with hospitals. As this happens, the income of these physicians becomes shifted into the hospital costs and makes hospitals appear to cost more.[3]

Whenever hospitals run ambulance services, costs may be shifted into their budgets without increasing the costs. Cost-shifting may occur when hospitals build parking garages, or doctors' office buildings. Cost-shifting rather than cost increasing is involved in the provision of ambulatory surgical units, to the extent that doctors may use such facilities rather than provide the services in their offices. Cost-shifting distorts the component of the health care dollar attributed to physicians. Since almost half of a physician's gross income is spent on overhead, it is misleading to say that physicians account for 20 percent of the health care dollar; only 10 percent really goes to them before taxes. If practice patterns should shift so that doctors dispense medications in their offices, for example, the portion of the health care dollar going to physicians would then seem to increase considerably; but physician before-tax income might not actually change at all.

So we have to admit we can only approximate the gross national product, and then only guess how much is attributable to hospitals, net of cost-shifting. However, no one seems likely to dispute the widely uttered statement that hospital costs are rising faster than the cost of living.

Having thus narrowed our focus to causes of hospital cost escalation exclusive of general inflation and mere cost-shifting, what are the options? Those most businessmen would mention would be:

---

3. Cost shifting is a two-way street. The recent threat of federal cost caps has stimulated a conversion of salaried hospital-based physicians back to private practice. Deferred or accelerated maintenance is another variant of cost shifting, in which costs shift to a different year.

1. Increased profits
2. Decreased employee productivity
3. Decreased management performance
4. Shifting to a more expensive line of service products.

The cost of living rose 7 percent last year, and average hospital room charges rose 11 percent. How much of that $5 billion went for each of the four causes we postulate? What is wrong with our powers of analysis when only four highly unflattering explanations can be found for a phenomenon we deeply hope has some legitimate explanation?

The mathematics and source data necessary to answer the query are beyond the resources of a mere physician; a full-scale Ph.D. dissertation would be required by a quantitative mind. But how to go about answering the query is clear enough:

1. The daily room charge is a very poor tool to use in judging hospital costs (see Chapter 7, "A Primer from the Trustees").
2. The residual value of hospital capital assets is the profit (see Chapter 12, "Building Mrs. O'Leary's Hospital").
3. And the other issues are considered in the next two chapters. On balance, how do hospitals emerge from the appraisal?

Where Does All the Money Go?

Changes which have taken place in the activities conducted within hospitals help to shed some light on the escalation of hospital costs, changes which go beyond mere numbers. Presumably an accountant could issue paychecks by the thousands, or a purchasing agent could buy supplies by the ton, without either one of them having any good explanation for the increase in size and number of paychecks and purchase orders. It is when we look up from the ledger books that a doctor may offer some help in public understanding of what is costing more in hospitals.

We will discuss eleven factors in the cost escalation. Three have been blamed but probably do not really count for much, three have had a real impact on costs but are nevertheless highly desirable, three are extremely expensive and have no redeeming value, and two are partly desirable, partly undesirable. We begin with the three factors which have been unfairly blamed for costs: the advances of science, the aging of the population, and medically unnecessary care.

THE COST OF NEW TECHNOLOGY

We have heard so much about CAT Scanners, cobalt radio therapy units, and other big-ticket equipment that the idea is growing that medical advances always add to the cost of medical care. But there are cost-effective medical advances, too. Think of smallpox vaccination, which has almost eradicated the disease from the whole world. In a few years, even the cost of vaccination will disappear as we stop protecting against a nonexistent disease. Think of the conquest of tuberculosis, which has changed from the commonest American cause of death to a rarity in one generation. All of those TB sanatoria are now closed or changed to other purposes because of medication which may cost as little as fifteen dollars a case, if you can find a case. Let's stop wringing our hands about the over-medicated population long enough to remember that tranquilizers have been almost as effective in closing psychiatric hospitals as isoniazid was with TB sanatoria. Does no one remember untreated pernicious anemia? Or diabetes before insulin? Or President Coolidge's son who died of an infected blister?

What sort of short national memory forgets President Roosevelt's case of polio, a disease which is just about extinct because of a five-dollar vaccine? Someone in pursuit of a Ph.D. might want to add up the cost effectiveness of all medical advances, with or without CAT Scans. To a doctor, such an accounting exercise is an insult. This book will drop the subject right here with a declaration: Medical technology in the past thirty years has clearly lived within its own budget, the cost-effective advances paying for the cost-augmenting ones.

The cost effectiveness of new technology presents itself in a wide spectrum of situations. There are a few new treatments, like cardiac surgery and chronic renal dialysis, which are just plain expensive. More commonly, the technological advance is not devastatingly expensive for the individual but is expensive for society or insurance companies when its use is widespread. Breast

X-rays for breast cancer are an example. There is little doubt that a breast X-ray (mammogram) is capable of detecting a cancer one or two years earlier than it can be felt as a lump; there is not much dispute that the incidence of involved lymph nodes is lower in cancers detected by this technique, and hence that the survival rate is greater. Unfortunately, a great many expensive X-rays must be taken to save one woman's life, and there is no way of knowing beforehand which woman that will be. Women over age fifty who have a yearly mammogram are spending close to fifty thousand dollars for each woman among them whose life is saved. Women who can afford it think this is very worthwhile, and insurance helps more women to afford it. The insurance company may not be able to afford it, however. In this sort of dilemma the claim that health care is a right is answered by the reply that technology is bankrupting the country. As in a country auction, if you are willing to pay fifty thousand, the auctioneer will next ask if you are willing to go to a hundred.

A similar question arises over the matter of preoperative testing. If it seems silly to obtain an electrocardiogram on every young man who is about to have his hernia repaired, the anaesthesiologist will reply that his malpractice insurance company will not permit him to take the risk of giving anaesthesia without the protection of obtaining a preoperative cardiogram on everyone. In this sense, society as a whole is deciding on the cost of repairing a hernia, and society is leaning heavily on the insurance mechanism to pay for its decisions.

But these things do change. It once would have been considered gross negligence to fail to obtain a Wasserman test at the time of admission of every single patient. However, syphilis has become so rare and the consequences of having undetected syphilis so minor that most patients no longer are given the Wasserman. Technology eventually catches up with its own costs, and eventually pays its own way.

MEDICALLY UNNECESSARY CARE

Let's make a disarming admission.

There possibly are a few patients admitted to hospitals without adequate medical justification. There could be a certain amount of unnecessary surgery. A certain number of patients may stay in the hospital longer than they should, and quite a few patients experience internal delays in service which, retrospectively, might have been avoided. But stop. All of these issues are minor, and they are diminishing. Wasteful medical uses of hospital beds are certainly not increasing in extent, as they would if that would explain cost escalations in excess of the cost of living. Consider: The average length of stay in hospitals has historically decreased from 20 days per admission in the year 1900 to less than nine days, at present. More precisely, days of hospitalization per thousand Blue Cross subscribers in Philadelphia, for example, have declined 30 percent between 1970 and 1978.

Professional Standards Review Organizations, or PSROs (see Chapter 21), have searched for medically unnecessary admissions over the whole United States, and their efforts have been criticized by the Office of Program Evaluation as possibly indicating that medically unnecessary admissions may be so infrequent that the cost of $10 per case to search for them is itself a little hard to justify. Using the 1978 average cost per hospitalization of about $1,600, the $10 would only be justified if one admission in 160 turned out to be unnecessary. As far as surgery is concerned, it is ironic that so much congressional and other attention has been turned to the one area of medical care ordinarily advised by one doctor and performed by a second. It can only be a matter of time before the second opinion programs on the necessity of surgery will have to defend their own costs, and probably acquire a certain notoriety for occasionally stimulating requests for third, fourth, and fifth opinions. Meanwhile, the public is speaking its real mind about second opinions: As judged by the lack of response, second opinions are just too much bother.

Delays in hospital discharge are indeed a problem. PSRO review experience in most areas shows that the most important cause of delayed discharge from a hospital is the unavailability of a suitable alternative place to convalesce. State Medical Assistance programs often fail to provide a reimbursement level adequate to cover nursing home costs, so the homes will not accept patients covered by Medical Assistance. The State of New Jersey attempted to correct this problem recently by mandating that nursing homes accept a quota of medical assistance patients. Since such a procedure could only take place if the charges of other patients were raised to subsidize it, the process might well make nursing homes too expensive for anyone to afford. At the same time, one must reluctantly sympathize with bureaucrats who are given only a limited budget by the legislature, and one must sympathize in turn with the legislature fearing to increase taxes. Even with grossly inadequate payment schedules, many state budgets for state-funded chronic care are larger than their budgets for acute care.

So a certain number of patients possibly do stay too long in the hospital, and the productivity of hospitals is somewhat decreased by seemingly avoidable internal delays. But a central point has to be hammered. One cannot possibly blame the escalation of hospital costs on excess utilization, when it is so easy to demonstrate that hospital use has steadily and markedly declined during the period we are talking about. Utilization has gone down, costs have gone up.

POPULATION TRENDS

While it is clear that age-corrected population groups are experiencing fewer days of hospital care than formerly, the entire population is becoming more elderly. Patients eligible for Medicare are increasing at a rate of 5 percent a year. Older persons experience more illness, hospitalization, and medical expense. The average length of stay of Medicare patients is approximately ten days per admission, while the younger patients on Medical Assistance (Medicaid) stay only about five days in the hospital for their less serious illnesses. Roughly 40 percent of acute hospital beds are now filled with Medicare patients, and the proportion is certain to increase as the population curve matures. Anne Somers has described the even more exaggerated situation in Sweden. In that country, 15 percent of the hospital beds are filled with patients above the age of eighty, and extrapolation of existing trends leads to the prediction that within twenty-five years, 35 percent of Swedish hospital beds will be occupied by patients over the age of eighty.

The cost implications of such population trends are serious. If one allows his mind to dwell on the year 2025, it becomes positively appalling to calculate the American health care costs which will be related to the post-World War II baby boom reaching the age of eighty. Major political upheavals lurk within such distortions of the shape of the population pyramid. The nature of the practice of medicine is certainly destined to be changed as society changes its views about health care as a right, and even the right to life.

But important as the population issue is clearly destined to become, it does not suffiice to explain very much of our past and present hospital cost explosion. Two examples may be convincing.

The price of a private hospital room in 1925 was $5 per day; the price of a new Buick was $700. By 1978, a private room had increased to perhaps $200, while a Buick could be bought for $7,000; a tenfold increase in the car compared with a fortyfold increase in the room. An elderly patient may use the hospital room more often and for longer periods than a young patient, but aging of the population has nothing to do with the rate increase.

Second example. While Blue Cross plans do offer "over 65-Specials" (or supplemental insurance), the great bulk of their subscribers are under the age of sixty-five. After that age, retirement from the work force combined with the availability of Medicare tends to isolate Blue Cross from the health costs of the aging population. Accepting a certain imperfection in the statistical method, one can gain some insight into the health costs of Americans still young enough to be in the work force. The 1979 annual report of Philadelphia Blue Cross demonstrates that this population group has had an increase in the inpatient claim cost per subscriber[4] as follows:

YEAR	INPATIENT COST PER SUBSCRIBER
1974	$100
1975	120
1976	138
1977	155
1978	170

4. A report by an insurance company might be misleading if its share of the total cost of hospitalization should be changing. The inpatient coverage of Blue Cross is so comprehensive, however, that this flaw is almost certainly not present in the figures cited. Note also that decreased usage within fixed costs might well increase unit prices, but the overall cost to the community will not increase. Therefore, the insurance premium, or the total cost (as a portion of gross national product) will not rise. Fixed and variable costing also will not explain a rise in the total subscribers cost.

It is easy enough to see the steady, recent increase in claim cost per subscriber, per year. The true significance of these figures is that they took place over a period of time when days of hospitalization were significantly decreasing, and they took place in a group of subscribers largely cut off at age sixty-four. Neither the amount of hospitalization nor the aging of the population can explain these increases. What is increasing is the price.

It is clear that we are getting a costlier hospital product. Costliness in excess of inflation cannot be explained by inflation (of course), nor can it be explained by aging of the population. Since hospitalization is steadily and appreciably decreasing, cost inflation cannot be explained by excessive hospitalization.

The United States Senate was perplexed by the escalation of hospital costs, and authorized a study (S. Res. 71) which appeared in December 1978 as a report of the Senate Committee on Governmental Affairs. There, the problem is stated:

> What accounts for the spiraling costs of hospitals? Wage and other expenses have increased, but they are only a fraction of the overall escalation. For example, had hospital workers earnings risen only as fast as those of private non-farm production workers, the annual rate of increase of hospital cost per patient day from 1950 to 1975 would have been reduced from 9.9, to 8.8 percent. Between 1967 and 1977, above-average increases in hospital worker's earnings have been responsible for only about one-fourth of the increases in hospital costs in excess of general price increases, and price increases for materials, equipment and utilities also accounted for a relatively small proportion of the total cost escalation. Thus neither wage nor price increases are the major factor here.

and the analysis is given:

> Rather, about three-fourths of this increase is due to the expansions of resources used for each day of care provided. In other words, more equipment and possibly greater availability of service, combined with perhaps less efficient use of what exists, account for most of the relatively excessive inflation of hospital costs.

It is heartening to see that Senator Abraham Ribicoff, chairman, and the other senators on the Committee on Governmental Affairs subscribe to what they call the "true explanation," which is:

the existence of third-party subsidies and insurance, such that regardless of the nature of available information, patients tend to demand more complete and more sophisticated care than they would if faced with the full costs of treatment.

Let us restate the Senate report. The best available analysis seems to show that extensive health insurance and subsidy has been the cause of a hospital cost inflation which had the following relative components:

1. 50 percent of cost escalation due to inflation itself.
2. 12 percent due to upgrading of hospital wages in excess of inflation.
3. 38 percent due to hiring extra people, building new buildings, and purchasing more hard goods.

So much for costs. It is clear that the most urgent need is to examine whether the public is receiving appropriate value for its decision to create an insurance mechanism which causes more hospital employees to be hired, at higher wages, utilizing more hard goods, in larger, newer buildings. This book will attempt to be fair about it, but in a sense the effort is futile. As the senators said, more money is being spent than the public would have paid if faced with the full cost.

What the senators are describing is known in economics class as the moral hazard of insurance. The moral hazard is a central concern of this book, so please note.

THE CONTRIBUTION OF NATIONAL INFLATION
TO HOSPITAL INFLATION

A reader might be troubled by the difference between the rather low estimate of the contribution of general inflation to hospital cost escalation provided by the Senate Committee on Governmental Affairs (50 percent), and calculations of the American Hospital Association Office of Research Affairs that 66 percent of the rise in hospital expenses is caused by an increase in unit costs.

The central issue in the statistical argument is the base period from which the calculation is made. The Senate report was speaking of the hospital system of 1950 as the baseline. If any hospital were still practicing 1950 medicine in 1979, its costs would have risen in 29 years, but only 50 percent as much as costs have actually risen. The American Hospital Association calculation, on the other hand, is based on 1977 experience, and includes the inflation in price of a great many items which were introduced long after 1950, and likewise includes the wage escalation of new job categories added between 1950 and 1976. The first year a hospital buys a CAT Scanner, its cost is pure increase in "inputs" (or a pure "expansion of resources used"), but in every subsequent year the CAT Scanner usage is subject to inflation of wages, repairs, electricity, etc. Whether you regard the CAT Scanner inflation cost in its second year as part of general inflation or as part of the expansion of resource use will depend on what base year is employed to make the calculation. It will also depend on whether you believe the CAT Scanner was an "unnecessary addition" or a "normal accommodation to advancing practices." The Senate figure is a useful challenge to the hospital system to examine its advances since 1950, and justify them, while the American Hospital Association figure limits the argument to the 1976-77 advances.

Even if the advances can be justified in their historical context, they must be measured against the coming deluge of hospitalizable illnesses which will inexorably be produced by the aging of the population. We may have to consider a less opulent style of hospitalization in the future, just as a bachelor may drive a Porsche, but after he has children to support he finds he has to switch to a Chevrolet.

Our problem is that about a third of each year's cost increase is caused by innovation, whereupon each innovation is subject to inflation in future years. The effect over thirty years has been that the cumulative innovations cost more than the whole hospital we began with. It therefore becomes an urgent matter to examine the scientific and sociological history of hospitals in the past thirty years. For better or for worse, what has changed in hospitals?

THIRTY YEARS OF HOSPITAL INNOVATION

The Ex-Resident Society of the Pennsylvania Hospital[5] honors some distinguished ex-resident physician each year with the Jacob

5. One of my big problems is the concern that someone will imagine that "the" hospital that ate Chicago is some particular hospital in disguise, and will engage in a guessing game as to which one it is. The most obvious candidate for such speculation would be a hospital with which I happen to be associated. This is completely wrong. The Pennsylvania Hospital, which I love, just happens to provide some handy anecdotes. It happens to be my own hospital, and it happens to be the first and oldest in America.

Ehrenzeller Award, named after that first physician apprentice who served the hospital in 1772. Award recipients tend to be elderly (they might not be around the next year), and they tend to respond to their award with amusing recollections of old days at the hospital. Such occasions are a useful annual reminder that people have always got sick with much the same diseases, and often managed to recover without our present technology. The average life expectancy in 1900 was forty-six, today is seventy-two. Some diseases of the past (tuberculosis, typhoid, syphilis) have virtually disappeared, but the diseases of today were also present in the past. Award recipients are generally gracious about the changes which have occured in their lifespan, but it seems impossible to receive an Ehrenzeller award without offering a wry comment on the vast increase in the number of administrators. Indeed, it will probably be 1990 before an elderly ex-resident will be able to recall the existence of more than a single administrator-and-secretary during the bygone day of his internship. This same hospital in 1978 spent $5 million on ever-expanding administration functions.

In 1969, the hospital broke tradition and for the first time in 209 years, paid a salary to its interns. An intern physician now is paid $15,500 a year.

In 1973, the hospital discontinued its nursing school, and replaced the unpaid (and slightly browbeaten) student nurses with registered nurses paid $16,500 a year, plus some licensed practical nurses paid $13,200.

In 1940, there were four hundred patients in large open twenty-bed wards. Today, all buildings are air conditioned, and all beds are motor driven. All patients have television sets, telephones, and intercom systems to the nursing station.

The parking garage, which holds four hundred cars, was excessively large in 1970. Today, it is being augmented by another three-hundred-car garage because the attendants must post a "full" sign at the entrance by 8:30 A.M.

The hospital has an annual budget of $50 million. A million dollars a week. Something clearly costs a lot more than it used to. Somewhere, between the imprecision of after-dinner nostalgia and the misleading jargon of accounting aggregates, it should be possible to identify the concepts that have changed. After that, comes an assessment of the cost and value of changing the concepts.

THE WAGES OF HOSPITAL WORKERS

People feel uncomfortable talking about their incomes, so most people have only a hazy idea of the income of their acquaintances. Hospital wages have changed dramatically in the past twenty years, but gradually enough so that normal respect for privacy has obscured the significant changes in social position of hospital employees. This was allowed to go on unnoticed until 1976, when Martin Feldstein blew a whistle. Contrary to prevailing belief, cleaning people in hospitals were paid more than cleaning people in banks; hospital telephone operators were paid more than telephone operators in business; hospital nurses were paid more than industrial nurses. It is difficult to equate technically trained employees in one industry with technical fields in other industry, but the implication was plain. Where hospitals and other industries offered the same jobs, hospital employees were better paid; so the other hospital employees might well be overpaid also. The existence of pervasive health insurance constantly tempts the hospital personnel manager to play Santa Claus. The insurance term for this process of undermining normal price resistance is "moral hazard."

It would appear that the moral hazard factor of insurance has also relaxed normal vigilance against overstaffing. If one divides the number of employees by the number of average occupied beds, a ratio is obtained, known as employees per patient. Because hospitals have a certain amount of bed vacancy, a lower ratio can be described: employees per bed. Since employees concerned with the emergency room and ambulatory services are in no way related to beds, occupied or not, the ratios have some misleading features. But for what they are worth, the ratios have shown a steady rise in recent years:

YEAR	EMPLOYEES PER BED*
1970	2.29
1971	2.34
1972	2.37
1973	2.40
1974	2.46
1975	2.53
1976	2.61
1977	2.71
1978	2.78

*Because of vacancies, employees per *patient* are roughly 30 percent higher.

An interesting way to examine hospital staffing is to calculate the number of full-time employees (or equivalents) per 100 hospital admissions. According to the American Hospital Association they were:

YEAR	PERSONNEL PER 100 ADMISSIONS
1970	5.72
1973	5.81
1976	6.21
1978	6.50

By dividing 6.5 into 100, we see that each average hospital employee derives a yearly income equal to the revenue from 15 average patients. The statistic summons up an anecdote from my intern year in 1948. Dr. Leon Herman, the president of the medical staff at that time, on the eve of his retirement was able to boast to a goggle-eyed intern: "I make my living on fifteen patients a year. The rest can go to the ward." May Dr. Herman rest easy in his grave; his former intern now has to have two thousand active patients to make a decidedly less handsome income, and this is the universal experience of physicians today. The American Hospital Association provides additional statistics about the dramatic sociological change, demonstrating that physicians have increased in numbers somewhat, also.

YEAR	COMMUNITY HOSPITAL BEDS PER 100 NONFEDERAL ACTIVE PHYSICIANS
1968	338
1972	327
1976	324

To return to the present point, hospitals are hiring more employees and paying them more money. Some of the increase in salaries is the result of general inflation. Some results from an almost hysterical fear of unions by some hospital managements. Some comes from increases in the minimum wage law. Some from strong political pressure to increase the hiring and promotion of minority groups. Some of it is a one-shot conversion of unpaid student nurses, house physicians, and others in training to paid status. Some of it is a one-shot rectification of deplorable under-payment in the past. Some of it is a response to the increased requirements of new technology.

But all of it is exaggerated, accelerated, and made painless for hospital management by the so-called "moral hazard" or under-mining of normal price resistance which occurs because personnel costs can be passed through to insurance carriers and government third parties without pain to the patient. While every ingredient of the personnel explosion can be justified as a concept, no one would deny that the personnel explosion is greater than it would have been if insurance pass-through had not been the dominant form of hospital revenue. The Canadians have tried regulatory restraints; the consequence has been paralysis of medical progress. Mr. Nixon attempted a wage and price freeze. The result was a frenzied rush to get ahead of the game, to put on fat for the coming winter, and to penalize those hospitals with a conscience who were foolish enough to restrain themselves. Make no mistake about it. The moral hazard of third-party cost reimbursement is the villain. The hospital personnel manager is just trying to keep from drowning.

EVOLUTION OF HOSPITALS FROM LABOR-INTENSIVE TO CAPITAL-INTENSIVE

Since health care is a service industry, it suffers by comparison with production industries. Gains in productivity are easier to achieve if you are making hundreds of widgets: You simply gain economies of scale by making tens of thousands of widgets, and you make them with automated equipment. Since the rest of the economy is thus able to achieve gains in productivity, all service industries show up unfavorably in comparisons with general indices like the cost of living. Health care is no exception. It is common to hear that since two-thirds of a hospital bill ends up as wages, you aren't going to save much money until you fire some-body.

That situation is slowly changing. Although personnel costs have indeed skyrocketed, their proportion of the total hospital budget has dropped from 60 percent to 55 percent in the past five years.

If you subtract personnel costs, all other expenditures can be called either construction costs or purchases of supplies. Since the central complaint about hospitals is that their costs have risen faster than the cost of living, we can here ignore such mundane supplies as food, heating fuel, and utilities. Hospitals seem to be building new buildings and buying new medical supplies at a fearsome rate. It could further be argued that the whole cost process is driven upward by advancing technological improvements in the delivery of health care. Partly so, no doubt about it.

But it seems to at least one medical observer that one powerful unnoticed drive behind new building programs and new equipment has been the attempt to apply capital-intensive management techniques to reducing the labor costs of hospitals. Perhaps the main need will be to defend the future institution against the "English disease" of disruptive union rules. Perhaps the goal of reducing the cost of medical care can be reached by using disposable supplies rather than sterilizing and reusing. Perhaps new steel window frames will not require painting, perhaps the maintenance cost of automatic elevators will be less than the cost of elevator operators.

Perhaps. But in the process of trying to rationalize administration, hospitals have had to reinvent some industrial wheels. Like others before them, hospital corporations have learned that employing computers forces you to hire more employees, rather than firing some, as you had imagined. Hospitals have learned the hard way that a capital-intensive innovation is not necessarily a labor-saving innovation. And further, labor-saving is not necessarily the same as cost saving.

Perhaps all of this seems like ungraciously second guessing the managers who are doing their best, and probably they are doing better than others could do with the same problems. It may be so. But candor requires observation that the attempts to increase the capitalization of hospitals have three unfortunate qualities:

1. They increase the power, prestige, and salary levels of the management team. In this sense, they might be a little self-serving.

2. They cause employee unrest and tend to increase invisible retraining costs. Indeed, they might even incite anti-technology sentiments among the unions.

3. Cost reimbursements present very few obstacles to purchases, building costs, or interest charges on borrowings.
Therefore, the process of deciding to become capital-intensive
is seldom subjected to an agonizing balancing of costs in the
mind of the decision-maker. If the decision is wrong, too bad.

Taken all together, one is justified in having private doubts that
the drive toward capital-intensiveness in hospitals has been as
effective as it would have been if hospitals were operating in a
competitive environment without retrospective cost-plus reimbursement. It could, of course, be worse. Senator Edward Kennedy caused enactment of a National Center for Health Care
Technology, which may possibly lay the same dead hand on technology advance as has been evident in the Food and Drug Administration. Or worse still, the ultimate horror: The American public
might actually be stampeded into an antiscience, antigrowth,
antitechnology, antiproductivity madness. The English disease.

3

Across the Backyard Fence

"Hi, Jim."

"Hi, George. How's it going? Dorothy tells me you are writing a book about hospital costs."

"Yes, and about hospital charges. They're two different things."

"I don't get you."

"Well, for example, my aunt just spent two weeks in a hospital out West and sent me a copy of her bill. It was over $9,000. But the basic fact is that she isn't paying any of it, Medicare is. The size of her bill scares the wits out of her friends, but they all have Medicare, too, so it's pretty theoretical."

"How is she?"

"She's fine. Did just beautifully with an aneurysm that would have been completely hopeless twenty years ago."

"Wonderful. But you were going to explain the difference between costs and charges."

"Oh, yes. Well, her bill was $9,000 but the chances are that Medicare will only pay something like $6,000 which it says are the costs. The $3,000 difference is known as a contractual allowance. They have a contract, and the contract says they don't allow the full amount."

"Is that how it works? It really only costs $6,000?"

"God alone knows what it really costs. Using the Medicare accounting rules it appears to cost $6,000, but probably $4,200 of that is used to pay for the running of the institution, and only $1,800 is a direct cost of her illness."

"That really doesn't sound so good."

"Well, they couldn't operate on her in a cornfield. You have to have an institution."

"OK, OK, but $9,000 for something that only directly costs $1,800 is a little extreme, don't you think?"

"Indeed I do, that's why I wrote the book. If you want to make it look even worse, you might mention the cost of running Medicare, which has to be added to the total cost to society. I suppose it cost them $25 to process the claim, but if you wanted to be spectacular and talk fast, you might say it cost $2,000, bringing the total cost to $11,000."

"Great Scott. Now what's that all about?"

"I'm alluding to the fact that hospital costs are 45 percent of the total national health budget, and insurance administration is about 10 percent. But to be truthful, most of the cost of insurance is eaten up by a ton of small claims, not big ones like aneurysm repair."

"Say George, does anybody pay the whole $9,000?"

"Sure. If she didn't have insurance she would pay the whole $9,000. You almost have to have it to protect yourself."

"How do they decide how much discount you get?"

"It really isn't decided at all. Medicare, Medicaid, and Blue Cross don't even look at the patient's bill. They make lump-sum payments to the hospital every so often, and then at the end of the year they have a big auditing argument to settle up. They pay in bulk for all their patients at once. That's the reason nobody really knows what any one patient actually costs or what was actually paid."

"But isn't there some regular relationship between the charge and the cost?"

"If you're asking if there is a uniform markup, the answer is a loud 'No.' As a matter of fact, markups for some things can be 80 percent, while other items in the same hospital could be priced at less than cost."

"George, I've got to go, this stuff sounds pretty heavy."

"See you later, Jim. Stay well."

"Hey, wait a minute. I'm interested in your book, I really am. But what difference does it make to me, or to your aunt, for that matter, how the accountants juggle the hospital books? When we're sick we don't care much and when we're well we don't care at all."

"I suppose you don't care what your insurance premium is?"

"Let me tell you something, George. I don't even know what my health insurance premium is. And that's a pretty good feeling to have, right there."

"There was something called Section 1801 in the Medicare Act which said that Medicare wasn't supposed to interfere with or alter the practice of medicine. What a laugh. Medicare doesn't change the practice of medicine any more than the weather changes farming. If you don't care what it costs, at least you should care what it is."

"George, you doctors control the way hospitals are run. If you can't control your own shop, what can I do for you?"

"We control hospitals the way Christopher Columbus controlled the Atlantic Ocean. They aren't our hospitals. They are your hospitals. My hospital hasn't had a doctor on the Board of Trustees in two hundred years."

"OK, I'll run for election. How much does it pay?"

"Just exactly as much as I was paid as an intern."

"Well, OK, I guess I'll have to read your book."

"See that you do, Jim, or I'll throw crabgrass seed on your lawn."

4

What Does the Money Buy?

So much for an external description of rising hospital costs. It is now time to look at the same facts from the viewpoint of a human organization trying to adjust to violent changes in its basic premises.

In modern management theory it is a widely accepted belief that a good manager does not need to know very much about what he is managing. This unfortunate concept is sometimes even carried to the extreme of stating that to get mixed up in the minutiae of technology is a distracting handicap, since a manager's job is to identify and "maximize the bottom line." Each component of an organization is reducible to a numeric assessment of whatever you want that component to produce, balanced against some cost you wish it did not generate. Subtract one from the other and there you have the bottom line—don't bother yourself with all those technical details, and particularly don't bother to listen to lame excuses for nonperformance.

This sort of brusque intellectual expediency is quite frequently applied successfully to engineering, but we should have severe uneasiness when society applies the bottom line approach to medical care in a hospital. Simply speaking, the costs would seem to be salaries, supplies, and building construction. Costs are high, going higher. Eventually everybody dies in spite of the effort, anyway. Put hospitals on a budget and make them live within it. If they go beyond the budget, fire somebody.

In what follows, an attempt is made to identify some of the scientific, sociological, and political winds which are blowing up the costs of hospital care, causing people to be hired, supplies to be bought, buildings to be built—and the sick to be comforted. Let us see if we can make accounting serve the organization, and not the organization serve the accountants.

It is probable that the 1965 Congress and President Lyndon Johnson thought of Medicare and Medicaid in terms of permitting the poor and the elderly to have medical care which they would otherwise have had to go without for financial reasons. Such medically underserved people tended to concentrate in poor rural areas and in urban ghettos.

Unfortunately, it was inadequately recognized that physicians, nurses, and hospital employees were reluctant to live and work in urban ghettos or rural poverty areas. Those who would consent to work there were often suboptimal competitors in some sense: foreign-trained, perhaps, or supplementing a beginning practice in the suburbs, or stranded by the changes in neighborhoods. Hospitals long located in changing areas were particularly likely to be socially stranded; there were Protestant-run hospitals in totally Catholic neighborhoods, and Catholic hospitals in neighborhoods which were totally black. Such socially disrupted organizations were not well suited to readjust themselves to a sudden removal of the "financial barrier to health care access," and their potential clients were also not socially skillful. The situation adjusted slowly and expensively. If the suburban middle class had been given such free tickets to health care, the system could have adjusted suddenly and expensively, but it would have been a one-shot cost. However, even after fifteen years, the backlog of indigent care is still being worked off, and ghetto hospitals are still struggling in the process of costly upgrading to the suburban standard. Some expensive attempts have been made to accelerate the process, but mostly it is recognized that the sluggishness is due to the conservatism of sociological process.

The first wave of hospital construction in response to the 1965 laws concentrated on two features: air conditioning and the conversion of forty-bed wards to two-bed semiprivate rooms, the standard accommodation copied from the Blue Cross system of benefits. A hospital expected to make a profit on "private" (i.e., single-bed) rooms, expected to lose money on ward (i.e., forty-bed) patients, and to break even on semiprivate (i.e., two-bed) rooms. Nobody was going to make a profit at government expense, by golly, and of course the government pays its rightful share. In other words, Congress was buying nonprofit middle-class dignity, and that seemed to mean semiprivate rooms.

The results should have been predicted, but they weren't. Activists spread the good news of entitlement and rights to the indigents, and monitored to make sure that hospitals did not discriminate or, worse still, segregate. The mixing of patients from different races and social classes in a forty-bed ward had somehow been less abrasive than mixing them in pairs in a small room proved to be. Close confinement did not bring out the best in the anxious visiting families of the patients. It was no good. Experience with schools had taught the middle class how to flee to the suburbs for a little *de facto* segregation, and nobody had to draw anybody a picture.

So, three very expensive trends precipitated a second wave of hospital construction: empty beds in center city, waiting lists in the suburbs, and conversion of two-bed rooms into one-bed rooms. The distortion is unquestionably a very expensive one, and no doubt it could be curtailed by brute force. The empty beds could be closed, and competitors both nearby and suburban would rejoice. But such a process would mean:

1. The suburbs would be forced to enlarge their hospitals, since waiting lists will not be tolerated indefinitely. A new cost would then ensue.

2. The hospital beds to be closed would not merely be center-city beds, but would especially be beds in deteriorating areas. By this means, a federal program to remove the barriers to health care access in the ghettos would have resulted in closing the ghetto hospitals completely. This is no wild theory. Fourteen hospitals in the deteriorating areas of Brooklyn have already closed.

3. Forcible restraint of construction of single-bed rooms would freeze us into a posture which was bad planning in the first place.

Historically, two people had been put into a semiprivate room because hospitals wanted to reduce the price of private care at the same time that they wanted to restrain everyone from

demanding that price reduction. No one considers it reasonable
to sleep in a room with strangers when checking into a hotel.
That sort of thing went out in 1850. The plain fact is that the
1950–70 wave of semiprivate room construction was a dumb
idea, and the sooner we rectify the blunder the better.

MEDICINE TAKES TO THE HILLS

The architects of the Great Society had been shown by Michael
Harrington that there was rural as well as urban poverty. For rural
poverty read sharecroppers, migrant workers, and Appalachia.
The Medical Assistance programs established by the 1966 Title XIX
amendments to the Social Security Act provided funds for first-
class medical care for the rural unfortunates, providing they could
find it. Rural America had already been sprinkled with small
modern hospitals by the Hill–Burton legislation. Indeed, it is fair
to say that the little hospital is almost invariably the most modern
building in any small town you wish to visit. The hospital is often
the only institution in a small town with any glamour, the place
where the town ladies work as volunteers, the town worthies serve
as trustees, and the prettiest girls in high school become student
nurses. Out of such local pride grows enormous political lobbying
power for the American Hospital Association.

The construction of modern facilities, the infusion of large
amounts of federal hospital revenue through Medicare and
Medicaid, the political clout, the local pride, the interstate highway system, and the congestion of nearby suburban hospitals all
combined to raise the medical expectations of rural areas. Meanwhile, the cost-reimbursement system made it possible to reimburse the advanced training of many more specialists, who began
to consider favorably the idea of settling in exurbia. Given any kind
of decent school system for his kids, the move to the country was
decidedly tempting for a young newly trained specialist.

The effect of all of this was to undermine the old hierarchal
hospital pecking order and to set off a competition for new prestige
relationships. The old concept had been that because a hundred
medical school hospitals were the hubs of wheels constantly creating new knowledge, they received "tertiary care" referrals of the
most difficult cases from the larger "secondary care" community
hospitals who in turn received the moderately difficult cases from

primary care (i.e., little and rural) hospitals out at the ends of the spokes of the wheel. Problem cases would be referred toward the center, while new medical knowledge would percolate out in the opposite direction. The hierarchal organization of hospitals was patterned after the military hospital system, which was organized to administer first-aid triage near the fighting front, but to send back to base hospitals the more difficult cases. The military tradition helps to explain why the tertiary care referral centers, at the center, tend to expect to make decisions and expect obedience from the primary care hospitals on the firing line. Florence Nightingale devised this system for the Crimean War; every war tends to reinforce this pattern on the civilian medical community, while every long period of peace and prosperity tends to fragment it. It is surprising that so few were able to foretell that the advent of Medicare and Medicaid in 1965 would severely strain this hub-and-spokes pattern, and that competitors for medical prestige might well give the teaching hospitals a run for it. The dominance of the teaching hospitals can quite clearly be seen in retrospect to have depended heavily on their greater access to funds, as well as their large pools of indigent patients available for teaching purposes. Medical Assistance (Medicaid) eliminated the indigent wards, and the advent of easy federal money was a good equalizer of other things. Why send your patients to the Mayo Clinic when it is just as easy to hire the Mayo doctor and have him work right here?

It isn't as simple as that, of course, nor rapid, nor certain. But it is surely true that one of the invisible forces causing national medical care costs to rise is the steady broadening of the medical pyramid, with much less difference in quality of care existing between city and country as time goes on. However desirable such developments may be, a rapid commotion of a system will cause some waste. Inevitably there will be some overoptimistic construction, some unkept promises, some disappointed abandonments. As long as a system is in flux, there will be reorganization costs.

At some point however, the regional population becomes too thin to support a full-service local hospital system. The boundary between appropriate and inappropriate population density will depend on transportation, traditional trading patterns, the degree of local pride or conservatism, and historical happenstances.

Some towns will demand to have a cardiac surgeon if anyone else has one, while residents of other towns are more casual about hopping a plane to St. Louis. In my own area, there is an invisible sociological line running through Valley Forge, Pennsylvania. A man who lives to the south of that line regards himself and his neighbors as Philadelphia commuters. A hundred yards north of the invisible line, people mean Pottstown when they say they are going "to town," and they mean Reading when they say they are going to "the city." Going to Philadelphia is to them like going to Paris.

But, local color to one side, the medical boundaries are really a dynamic equilibrium between the expense of travel and the expense of subsidizing the local hospital. When it is your own money being spent on travel, but the government's money which subsidizes the local facility, it becomes pretty clear that the boundary is going to be shifted toward developing more local facilities. And that, dear reader, is one of many reasons medical care costs are rising faster than the cost of living. Whether total community health costs are raised by this process is a far more sophisticated question.

THE DESTRUCTION OF THE OSLER SYSTEM

In 1870 Dr. William Osler came to Philadelphia from his home in Canada, and started a system of "hands-on" medical education at the Philadelphia General Hospital, which at that time had a census of eight thousand patients. In 1970 the Philadelphia General Hospital (PGH) closed its doors and scattered the three hundred remaining patients. During those hundred years, the Osler system caused American medical education to flourish into undeniable world leadership, copied by most and envied by all. But the 1965 amendments to the Social Security Act unintentionally destroyed that system of training, and American medical education has floundered for 15 years trying to come to terms with the new environment. One cannot make omelets without breaking eggs, we are told. Whatever the ultimate educational accommodation of American medical education to its new constraints, the financial cost of the accommodation has so far been pretty staggering.

The Osler system was a set of trade-offs. The indigent patients got free care. The students, interns, and senior attending physicians provided the care without pay. The students and interns received their instruction from the attending physicians, and the attending physician enormously extended his prestige and experience by functioning at the narrow end of the consulting funnel. To give some idea of the educational experience available, in 1945 there were 2,400 autopsies performed at the PGH. (Today, there are very few hospitals which perform more than a hundred a year.) Routine morning rounds would consist of the professor and his assistants visiting the bedside of eighty patients. PGH's pool of clinical experience was enormous; most interns could expect to deliver over a hundred babies, and participate in hundreds of surgical procedures. Osler set the style for attitudes about the medical literature, which was very close to "we don't read books; we write books." In one address he intoned that "To practice without reading is to sail an uncharted sea. To read without practicing is never to set to sea at all."

The student nurses meanwhile worked for three years on the indigent wards to obtain their diplomas. The X-ray technicians worked a similar apprenticeship. And such was the system in two-thirds of the hospital beds in Philadelphia in 1945. A report of the Mayor's investigating commission in 1948 began: "Philadelphia can rightly be proud . . . "

Well, it was a two class system of medicine and it had to go. The affluent society could afford to give decent dignity to all its sick citizens, while the apprenticeship system was a relic of the exploitation of child labor. The system is gone, and it isn't coming back.

But we have pretended that the old rules still apply, when they don't. All patients are now "private" patients, and the upwardly mobile are particularly touchy about it. If Lyndon Johnson provided the money for first-class surgery, the patients were not about to have their surgery performed by an intern. Or their baby delivered by a medical student. Or the lump in the breast displayed to a gawking class. So there has been a retreat to the library and the classroom blackboard. "Grand Rounds" is now a quaintly anachronistic term for a lecture given by somebody from out of town in the new auditorium instead of presentation of an actual patient and his problems for the full staff to discuss. X-ray conferences are quite popular; Journal Club[1] is a central function.

Technicians have been hired to draw blood specimens, a function performed by house officers in the past. Indeed, blood counts and urinalyses were the shared responsibility of interns and students, but are now performed by the laboratory staff. There is an intravenous nurse, and a hyperalimentation team. As indeed there should be. If there is no charity there is no need to be charitable. Lyndon Johnson emancipated more slaves than Lincoln did. But it was expensive.

It is expensive also to hire full-time teachers, and to build auditoriums, and to pay the expenses of visiting lecturers. It is expensive to expand the library or connect it by computers to the National Library of Medicine in Bethesda. It is equally expensive to cut physicians off from the educational experience as soon as they finish their residencies and pass their board examinations, but that expense takes a long time to appear.

Technology in medicine has advanced at such a pace that a system of education which fails to extend throughout a medical career is going to waste much of the technology. The old system of walking the wards included all generations of doctors, a group who tend to develop a strong aversion to lectures after about ten years of them.

It is expensive to support a system which provides unlimited specialty and subspecialty training for years at a time while paying reasonable salaries to unlimited numbers of residents. It is true that nothing could be worse than setting federal quotas for specialist training and rationing the supply of specialists. England has done this, and has waiting lists of patients for elective surgery by the hundreds of thousands while their hospitals are 20 percent empty. But on the other hand, the present financial incentives of the cost-reimbursed hospitals must surely be tilting the equilibrium in the direction of too many specialists and too few primary care physicians. That's an expensive component of the rising cost of health care, too.

---

1. Recent reviews of the articles in the medical literature by Williamson of Johns Hopkins, among others, suggest that only 0.5% of articles drew conclusions which were clinically relevant and statistically warranted. Of the significantly important articles selected by eminent teams nominated by the National Institutes of Health, 73 percent were unretrievable through a normal library search. Correspondence between significant articles selected by the NIH experts and citations in three standard medical text books was less than 10 percent.

To a certain extent, the reimbursement system which supports hospital residents can be regarded as a form of hidden subsidy to medical schools. The residents often spend considerable time teaching medical students, and the teaching hospitals increasingly have entered into contracts with medical schools which provide house officer in-service training[2] programs. But probably the major benefit to medical schools is their ability to raise tuition to the medical students to a level higher than the students might otherwise be able to afford. Remember that many students now graduate with twenty- or thirty-thousand-dollar debts, which can partly be paid back out of residency salaries. Even when student loans are not required, there is no doubt that family reserves of the medical student can be spent down more confidently when an income is assured after four years, rather than eight or ten as used to be the case. There are a few Porsches in the hospital parking lots, it is true. But probably much of the typical resident salary is committed to paying, in one indirect way or another, for undergraduate medical education.

PUKING IN THE NURSE'S ARMS

All the world's a stage, we hear in *As You Like It,* where all the actors begin by puking in a nurse's arms, and later end their strange eventful histories in a "second childishness . . . sans teeth, sans eyes, sans taste, *sans* everything." . . . We might get along in life without doctors and hospitals, but it is hard to imagine getting along without nurses.

But don't push it too far, nurse. The nursing component of the medical care dollar is being observed by computers, the quality of bedside nursing is being noted by the patients, there are plenty of competitors for the nursing functions, your boss the hospital administrator regards you as his worst headache, and only the doctors are your friends. For the time being.

Innumerable paperback novelists have observed that student nurses and resident physicians have a natural affinity, even if gruff old surgeons and stiff old matrons might not. Propinquity and shared duties under stress gave some substance to the idea of affinity in the years when a student nurse lived three years in the

2. In-service training is on-the-job training. Naturally it is preferred to tuition.

hospital before she graduated, while a two-year internship was just that: two years within the walls. Today's intern calls himself a resident but usually does not reside in the hospital. And a nursing student now scarcely sees the inside of a hospital until after she has graduated. Both groups are mostly already married.

Like so many wrenching changes to our system, this one was not mandated by the Medicare Act, but it could not have happened without it. By 1965, the austerities of nursing training and widened employment opportunities for women had led to quite a nursing shortage. At first, the plentiful funding provided by the Great Society made the shortages more painful as prices were bid up. Compromises were made with traditional nursing standards, particularly the burdensome ones. A nurse no longer stood up when a doctor entered the room. Peer pressure urged them to stop wearing those funny hats and to start wearing pants. Perhaps more serious was the discontinuation of the practice of having the head nurse visit the patient in the company of the attending physician when he made his rounds. The patient's medical record in some hospitals was broken into two parts, his and hers, so that the nurse would not have to surrender the chart to the doctor when he needed it; the consequence was that neither one read what the other wrote.

Hospital management naturally had to take a look at what could be done to relieve the overworked nurse. Functions were examined. The telephone could be answered by a clerk, and the clerk could copy doctor's orders, file reports, tidy up the desk and run errands. Licensed practical nurses could make beds, give back rubs, carry bed pans and get puked on. A pharmacist could administer medications. A junior member of the administrative staff could make out schedules and supervise the scene. The registered nurse thus only really had to do—what?

As the nursing shortage was washed away by an ocean of federal money, the nurses have either been specialized into the technological revolution or they write progress notes about the patient. If you see five nurses, the chances are you will see two of them writing. Meanwhile, all of the new entrants into the health care delivery field who were induced into hospital careers by the nursing shortage are also round about the nursing floor somewhere, mostly doing former nursing tasks less well than nurses used to do them. The potential for jurisdictional union disputes between these occupational competitors is very real, and almost certain to escalate. It is a serious comment that the cost of medical care is going to have to go up to provide extra hospital bed capacity because of this problem. To provide backup for hospitals which are closed by strikes.

Since the issue is so serious, a moment should be taken to examine the sociology of nursing. It was a fiercely cherished goal of the leaders of the nursing profession to get nursing training out of the exploitative hospital and onto a university campus. The universities were pleased if money was forthcoming. The instructors developed new status as professors, the students were capable of being convinced that a degree is more valuable than a diploma, and the hospitals were persuaded to give up the students by the nursing care cost differential (*vide infra*) plus ample funds to hire licensed practical nurses. But everybody forgot something.

The student nurse might have been intimidated and exploited, but she knew that if she stuck it out she was looking up a ladder, each step of which might eventually make her vice-president in charge of nursing, with an office right next to the administrator himself.

The licensed practical nurse had no such dreams. Typically she came from a social minority and entered practical nurse training after she had finished rearing her own children. Starting her career at age forty-five, she had no illusions that there would be time to ascend the ladder through the officer class to the high command. She was stuck. Hard work would only get her a backache. What is more, she was supervised by a twenty-year-old girl, probably white, who had hardly been in a hospital until the day she was hired. The quality of bedside nursing usually thus became whatever the practical nurse felt like making it, since the young supervisor was often too intimidated to do anything but hide behind a pile of progress notes. Another escape from the difficult situation was to specialize in the mechanical technology of the Intensive Care Unit, or anaesthesiology. But obsolescence overtakes you pretty fast in today's technology, and so it's a chancy career, technology.

The nursing care cost differential. Now, there you really have something. Some say that in 1969 the Nixon administration compensated hospitals for the insistence of Congress that the hospital reimbursement formula be reduced to 100 percent of costs (from the original 102 percent, which was intended to give a little leeway for slippage). In any event, starting in 1969 the reimbursement formula decreed that Medicare would pay the hospitals 108.5% of their nursing care costs.

The theory was as follows. Elderly patients are sicker and more demanding than younger ones. As a consequence, on a mixed general-duty floor, the nurse will be spending proportionately more of her time in a room with an old person than in the other rooms with younger ones. It would seem to follow from this theory that Blue Cross ought to pay 92 percent of the nursing care costs for its patients, but that is certainly beyond the control of Medicare. So, Medicare reimburses the hospital $1.085 for its share of every dollar spent on nurses. Since Medicare patients fill about 40 percent of hospital beds, the general upshot is that the hospital gets back approximately $1.03 for every dollar it spends on nurses.

Most rational people would expect that if you are going to get back $1.03 for every dollar you spend on nurses, you will be prompted to spend more dollars on nurses. You will at least consider raising their salaries, and hiring more of them. You will likely prefer higher-paid registered nurses to licensed practical nurses, and you will certainly prefer licensed practicals to unpaid student nurses. While it is impossible to read the motivation in people's minds, a look at the combined five-year statistics (1972–77) in the 242 hospitals of Pennsylvania suggests that the financial stimulus was neither unnoticed nor unapplied:

	1972	1977	% CHANGE
Patient Days Served	15,452,000	15,733,000	+ 2%
Number of Registered Nurses	26,336	33,342	+26%
Number of Practical Nurses	10,397	12,035	+16%
Full-time Students	2,267	1,102	−51%

THE KNOWLEDGE AVALANCHE

Ever since World War II, the scientific research community has been turning out an avalanche of new discoveries. Never mind that the cause of cancer is still unknown. The mind of man simply cannot absorb information as fast as it is currently being produced, and indeed libraries cannot hold it all. The National Library of Medicine currently acquires 250,000 articles a month. No other library in the world can afford to own even a fraction of its collection.

There is, therefore, so much basic scientific information already in existence that the research and development community cannot keep up with producing all of the new medical technology which it is perfectly possible to produce. And the medical profession in turn has trouble assimilating and utilizing the avalanche of new medical technology as it pours forth. The pace of technological obsolescence is breathtaking. The cost of this scramble is very great.

No one would have it otherwise, but the internal strains on the medical system during this golden age of medicine are almost invariably reflected in an increase in costs. For example, malpractice insurance.

You can scarcely blame a patient for resenting the fact that he did not receive the benefit of a piece of knowledge which had been quite lucidly laid out in an article in the medical literature. On the other hand, he cannot expect his doctor to read and remember 3 million articles a year. So we specialize, and refer cases to other specialists. Medical costs rise. The public resents the fact that there are no family doctors anymore.

The Food and Drug Administration tries to slow down the pace of new drug introductions by raising the cost and requirements of approval. So, American doctors are tortured at medical conventions by doctors with foreign accents who describe the splendid results they have been achieving abroad with drugs which American doctors are forbidden to use. Clinical drug research goes into foreign exile, and the cash flow shifts to drug companies headquartered in Switzerland. Bootleg drugs come in from Canada. American doctors purport to be doing clinical drug research when all they are really doing is building practices with advance possession of new pharmaceuticals.

Each new test or device is seized by the resident house physicians and applied in all directions, searching for the limits of usefulness. By the time the reasonable best use is defined, the test or device may well have been made obsolete by a new one. It would be preposterous to block the introduction of these new advances although we will probably see it tried. What is needed is

some modification of the reimbursement system so that conscious-
ness of true costs can enter the equation of whether a new advance
is worth its costs, or whether the old method would be good
enough. Right here is one of the two major risks in any proposal to
extend universal national health insurance to high risk ("catastrophic cost") medical financial disasters. The research and development world has a breathtaking ability to produce technology
of all sorts, great and small. Just pass a law saying you will pay for
things that are expensive—whatever the cost—and they will become expensive, all right. And then try to find a politician who will
say that the benefit once given should be taken away, or limited to
the constituents of some other congressional district.

If there is more to read and learn, more time must be spent
learning it. Residency training must take more years. The doctor in
practice must go to more conventions, read more books, take more
courses, pass examinations wearing bifocals. More time for education means less time for practice, hence higher fees. It probably
also means earlier retirement, so more medical students are
needed.

And smart medical students, not just ordinary well-intentioned
ones. The appalling crush of applicants for medical schools has had
the effect of raising intellectual standards for admission to the very
highest percentile of testing scores, and encouraging workaholics
to boot. Is this level of talent necessary for the current practice of
medicine? No, but it is barely good enough for the incredible
implicit demands of a lifetime of scientific revisionism, innovation,
and coping with professional change. If anyone can cope with the
knowledge explosion, it should be these kids. But they can't. They
will have their share of malpractice suits.

FROZEN ORGANIZATIONAL SYSTEMS

The theme we have been pursuing for the moment is that much
of the rising cost of medical care is ultimately traceable to the costly
process of adjusting to violent change. Change in medical education, change in the system of medical charity, change in the
geographic locus and breadth of medical quality, change in the
nursing profession, and change in science and technology. The
further theme is sounded that all of this change was either caused

or greatly accelerated by quirks and clauses in the third-party (or government-funded) reimbursement system. Some subsidies like the nursing cost differential were direct, while some others were pleasant discoveries of what was possible within the rules (see Chapter Eight, "Further Subsidies") and mostly they all imposed moral hazard on the hospitals to expand activities previously constrained by cost limitations.

It is important to note, however, that still other costs have been generated by inflexibility imposed on the system by the same reimbursement process. Certain programs become inappropriately frozen in place when money is unlimited for established systems but unavailable for innovative ones. Generous payment programs inevitably provoke strict rules to limit their scope. As control of the payment system thereby gets more remote from the arena of medical decision-making, the payment system pays less attention to medical care and more attention to its own imperatives. The resulting bottom-line approach leads to one central sin: Expediency. An example of where expediency leads you was the reply of John Maynard Keynes to the concern that the Social Security system would eventually go bankrupt: In the long run, we are all dead.

Hospitals have become locked into an acute care definition of their function; it seems probable that poor reimbursement for nursing home care has something to do with this. Indeed, hospitals even fear the concept of "swing beds," by which beds might for a time serve a nursing home function and at other times revert to acute care; there are reimbursement uncertainties. On the other hand, ambulatory service reimbursement is so insulated from cost competition that many hospitals are even expanding out-patient activities for which their overhead costs are highly unsuitable. For such functions, what is most efficient is not a medical department store, but rather a medical shopping center.

Internally in the hospital organizational reporting system, the pattern of departments has been frozen by the Medicare step-down[3] accounting process. A whole industry has grown up selling computer programs for three-and four-cycle step-downs, and another industry sells assistance in maximizing hospital depreciation. It is

3. A technical term, deriving from the appearance to a flight of stairs on the departmental cost reports which are required by Medicare.

almost unthinkable that hospitals could afford to restructure their departments so that the nurse reported to the doctor instead of to the vice-president of nursing. The reimbursement programs have ballooned the bureaucracy of hospitals to the point where the situation cries out for some decentralization. But at the same time, the hospitals would lose reimbursement if the indirect costs were apportioned in any way other than the present mysterious one, and they aren't about to have that.

If the situation is capable of a brief summary it is this: The reimbursement mechanisms have frozen the table of organization at the same time that they have imposed momentous changes on the system. It is a very expensive combination of effects.

EMPLOYEES IN THE HOSPITALS OF PENNSYLVANIA 1972–77*

	1972	1977	CHANGE NUMBERS	%
Physicians & Dentists	2,016	2,234	+ 218	(+10)
Registered Nurses	26,336	33,342	+ 7,006	(+26)
Licensed Practical Nurses	10,397	12,035	+ 1,638	(+16)
All Other Salaried Employees	82,802	103,980	+17,078	(+20)
Total Full-time Personnel	125,551	151,591	+26,040	(+21)
Medical & Dental Residents	3,502	4,187	+ 685	(+20)
All other Trainees	2,267	1,102	− 1,165	(−51)

*Source: Hospital Association of Pennsylvania

5

John Gromadsky's Brother

The bulky man waited for a traffic light to change, and when the heavy rush hour traffic stopped, he lumbered across. He was wearing a brown suit which fit him well enough, but somehow he looked uncomfortable in it. For one thing, he didn't have any neck. His head seemed to rise directly from his shoulders, and although he was well over six feet tall he looked short and squat.

The sidewalk on the other side was busy with a rush hour crowd hurrying to work in neighboring buildings, and the big man waited to approach the ornately cast bronze doors directly in front of him. The entrance was very large, and the building rose at least thirty floors above it. He pushed through the heavy door and from a crowded, noisy, hot outside world he walked into a very empty, very cool, very spacious lobby. Class. Real class. From behind a reception desk, a smiling white-haired security guard came forward.

"Can I help you sir?"

"Got a meeting. Thirty-four, forty-two."

The guard returned to his station and looked in his appointment book. He nodded. "Mr. O'Toole?"

"Naw," said the big man, "Anderson."

"Yes sir," said the guard, checking off his list and noting the time. "Please follow me. The elevators to the executive floor are down this corridor and then through the archway into the new building." The guard led the way, pushed the "up" button, and backed away with a warm smile.

"Just push the button for the thirty-fourth floor. When you get to the floor, just tell the receptionist that you have an appointment with Mr. Gerkenheimer. She'll just show you to his office. And I'll just send Mr. O'Toole up as soon as he arrives."

Anderson entered the carpeted, walnut-paneled elevator which whisked him upward rapidly and silently. The elevator stopped suddenly with a soft ring of a bell. It was only the thirteenth floor. Two clean-cut men with shiny red faces entered the elevator, the arrival of which had evidently interrupted an anecdote.

The two new passengers were absorbed in their story and ignored Anderson, who had backed up in the elevator until he hit its wall with a clatter. ". . . So then the sailor says: Well, all I can say is that when you go to bed with one of those guys, you get considerably more than just a good night's sleep!" The two men guffawed loudly, then grinned and settled into silence to wait for their floor. They could see that the button for the top floor had been pushed, so it was clear that all three passengers were going to get off on the same floor. The two jokesters made an elaborate ceremony of letting Anderson leave the elevator first. "After you, sir."

The blonde receptionist behind the desk had been alerted by the security guard. She rose to greet Anderson and led him to the president's office. Leading visitors down the hall was obviously one of her special talents, and Anderson enjoyed the experience. The history of this lady's employment had been that the president had told the personnel office to get someone to keep the union customers happy while they waited. In this, she had been a smashing success.

They went past the president's two real secretaries, who barely glanced up from their phone conversations. The two jokesters from the elevator lingered when they saw that Anderson was part of the meeting they were going to, so that the president could greet Anderson, ask him if he wanted a cup of coffee, and indicate that their meeting would take place on the two sofas at right angles in one corner of the room. Through the large windows was a magnificent view of the city and the surrounding mountains.

"The guard called from downstairs and said Mr. O'Toole has just come in. He'll be right up. This is Mr. Rial and Mr. Rogers, our two top marketing vice-presidents." Uncomfortable as he was, Anderson knew what to do next. His handshake nearly brought the two jokers to their knees. The president, immaculately tailored and manicured, killed time with chitchat. "Did you have any trouble parking your car?"

"Well, it's a new car so I put it in the garage across the street", replied Anderson, not knowing what he should say next. Mr. Gerkenheimer, the president, had the same worry, but more practice. "What kind of car did you buy?" he asked.

"It's a Buick Electra."

"Well, well," said Gerkenheimer, "I would think a union vice-president was entitled to a Cadillac."

Anderson nodded. "The membership don't like it if you live, you know, too high. Anyway," he paused, "a Buick is just as comfortable."

Gerkenheimer was about to give his views on the merits of various automobiles when Mr. O'Toole strode quickly and confidently into the room. A small elderly man, he spoke in startlingly loud and confident tones, and he looked brisk and domineering. "Good morning, Gerkenheimer. Why don't you get a real office instead of this boudoir you have here?"

Both men chuckled at this pleasantry, although both of them realized that it was the opening salvo of a contest, just as the office itself was designed to intimidate. Gerkenheimer, practiced in such matters, tended to pursue an elaborate ritual of courtesy in a smooth smiling mellifluous manner.

"Mr. O'Toole, you are very welcome to our little nook. We have to keep up with the competition, you know, from the other insurance companies that are equally anxious to have your union's business. And, for your own special convenience, the carpets in this room are fireproof. Just feel free to grind your cigar ashes into the rug."

Anderson and the two marketing men kept straight faces and tried to become invisible. Gerkenheimer and O'Toole both seemed pleased with the score on the opening exchange.

O'Toole now took charge of the meeting. "All right," he said, "let's get down to business. Let's see if you can earn your big salary and make our union membership a little happier with your health insurance."

The insurance company president responded, "My marketing people tell me that you have done such a good job in collective bargaining on behalf of your union members that the health trust fund now is building up a surplus. I assume you have come here to add one of our fine products to the package you have already been wise enough to select." He could see out of the corner of his eye that his marketing vice-presidents were trying to signal that something was wrong. But he had no doubt he was equal to the problem whatever it was.

"Well, yes," said O'Toole. "The health trust fund has got a little extra money in it. Not all employers are as tightfisted as the insurance companies."

Gerkenheimer got the message. His company wasn't unionized, but he wasn't going to let union customers pressure him into anything like that. So he hurried on to other subjects, although as he spoke, he could see that the marketing men were agitated about something else. The more the president talked, the more they squirmed. "Well maybe it's about time your union got our Major Medical package."

"We already got it," growled the union president.

"Well, how about the Excess Major Medical? It covers you up to a million dollars per lifetime?" O'Toole brushed him off with a wave of his hand.

"I see. Well, our Dental Plan is proving to be extremely popular". A disdainful look on O'Toole's face told him the union had that one, too.

"Vision Care is a dandy. The ophthalmologists had a fit when we included benefits for optometrists in the Vision Care package. As a matter of fact, the optometrists invented that one." O'Toole grinned, and showed where things stood on the Vision Care product. They had it.

At this point one of the marketing men thought he had better speak up. "They already have the Second Opinion Option, too, and the Ambulatory Services Rider," he said. "And last year they picked up the Preventive Care Package along with the Prescription Drug Prepayment Program."

"Well, I see," said Gerkenheimer, "you seem to have used up our whole bag of tricks. We're going to have to go back to the drawing board in the New Products Division."

"How about cancer?" asked O'Toole. "John Gromadsky's brother has cancer." At this, the insurance man's brow furrowed.

"Well, you know, we have the feeling that it isn't a good thing to pick out one disease and give benefits to someone who has that disease, which makes us deny the same benefit services to someone else just because he had tuberculosis instead of cancer. We have enough trouble telling if the service was rendered. For God's sake don't make us check out the accuracy of the diagnosis. What if the doctor had the wrong diagnosis for your brother?''

"Not my brother, John Gromadsky's brother. He's with the International."

"It's the same thing," Gerkenheimer impatiently went on. "We would be very willing to cover injections and X-ray treatments or whatever services the man needs, but please don't ask us to limit benefits to a single diagnosis. Give him Visiting Nurses, or back rubs, or things like that." At this moment to everyone's surprise, Anderson leaned forward and made his contribution to the issue.

"John Gromadsky's brother takes pills," he said. Gerkenheimer, who had been pushed a little too far by all this, shook his head and raised his voice.

"Now, listen, that's just silly. How can we administer a claims department if we have benefit packages that say we pay for pills if the patient has cancer? How do we know the patient has cancer? Do you realize it costs $6.39 every time we process a claim? Do you want to pay $6.40 for an aspirin? Don't you know that with the policy coverage you already have, it is inconceivable that a cancer patient would have anything at all that we don't already cover?"

Anderson looked uncomfortable at the tirade he had triggered. The marketing men, beginning to worry that their boss was going to lose the customer, started looking for an opportunity to tell a dirty joke to break up the tension. Mr. O'Toole was annoyed that he was getting out of his depth and had lost control of the conversation. So he stood up and started for the door. Over his shoulder he delivered his last, final, non-negotiable position. "Let's put it this way," he said. "You start with John Gromadsky's brother, and take it backwards from there. I'll see you guys later. I've got to go."

6

The Muddle of Hidden Subsidies

Third-parties (health insurance and government health programs) are thought to cover 88 percent of American individuals in 1979, and 94 percent of families to some degree. Coverage of the total health costs of the country (9.1 percent of the Gross National Product) however, varies from including only a part of hospitalization costs for a limited period of time to including every conceivable medical, dental, drug, appliance and nursing cost. Hospitalization for acute illnesses is the most usual benefit provided to almost everyone, with the consequence that in-patient acute hospital revenues are usually derived from third-party sources to a degree over 90 percent. The hospitals' financial health depends principally on their local third-party environment, with their losses mostly depending on their management of the small but precarious mixture of cash payments, bad debts and charity. Their central problem revolves around their inability to generate a profit on government-sponsored patients; in some parts of the country, Blue Cross patients must be added to the group from which no surpluses can be generated to cover other losses. On a nationwide basis, Blue Cross covers about half of the non-government patients but regions of the country vary enormously in the local proportion. Since Philadelphia Blue Cross is overwhelmingly predominant in its area, the problem is far worse for hospitals in Philadelphia than almost anywhere else. That is the major reason this book originates in Philadelphia. All hospitals have the same problem to some degree, but Philadelphia shows where it is leading.

We divide hospital revenues, therefore, into two general categories, the retrospective cost-reimbursement third-parties

(Medicare, Medicaid and Blue Cross), and the cost-plus-profit sources (commercial health insurance and self-pay).

1. *Medicare*, created in 1965 as Title XVIII of the Social Security Act, covers just about every citizen who has reached the sixty-fifth birthday, plus a few disabled younger persons, less a few older ones covered by the Railroad Retirement Act and other minor exclusions. Medicare is divided into Part A, which reimburses hospitals at cost, and Part B which pays doctors and out-patient services their charges. Whatever its population coverage, the financial impact of Medicare is disproportionately great because of the increased illness experience of the elderly (terminating, of course, in 100 percent mortality). The number of persons reaching age 65 is now increasing 5 percent per year. Medicare carries a deductible and coinsurance feature to involve the patients in a sense of responsibility for their costs, but sometimes this leads to bad debts which are then reimbursable. A great many persons have purchased supplemental insurance (i.e., "over-65-Specials") to cover these "gaps" in coverage; the effect of such supplemental insurance obviously defeats the usage restraints of deductibles and coinsurance, so it is a type of insurance which is difficult to defend as a concept. It is also difficult to challenge the freedom of people to respond to their problems with such supplemental insurance, although there is such widespread ignorance of the terms of Medicare that an education program might well be in order.[1]

2. *Medicaid* for the indigents became Title XIX of the Social Security Act in 1966, but there are appreciable differences between Medicaid and Medicare. The Medicare program is directly financed out of the Social Security Trust Fund, while Medicaid is a federal 50 percent matching program. The federal half of the Medicaid money comes from tax revenues and is administered by the states in their welfare programs. A separate agency of HEW supervised the program at first, but so much bureaucratic infighting took place that the Medicare and Medicaid programs were consolidated in the Health Care Financing Administration

---

1. Some insurance commissioners, on the other hand, have refused to allow premiums of "over-65-Special" policies to rise to a break-even level. The effect is to force a subsidy from other policy-holders. As with gasoline rationing, the seller loses his enthusiasm to sell the product when its price is artifically held down.

(HCFA). The problems were alleviated somewhat by this reorganization, but Medicaid continues to be difficult to administer because of its different source of federal revenue, and the need to yield to the prerogatives of 49 different state welfare agencies (Arizona never implemented a Medicaid program). The federal government would obviously like to make the program more manageable by taking it over, but fears the prospect of providing the remaining 50 percent of the funds. The states have lately become the most powerful and effective lobbyists in Washington, and the state bureaucracies which would be threatened by a federal takeover are strongly urging the advantages of local administration. If one cuts through the cross-accusations of incompetence, waste, and confusion of authority, there is one central truth about Medicaid: The states cannot afford to supply their 50 percent of the money, and unlike the Federal Treasury, cannot print money. The state administrators of the Medicaid programs have thus been presented with the problem of living up to program mandates without being given the money to do so. However sympathetic one may be with their impossible task, the record of corner-cutting and expediency has created a strong antagonism among all groups who have had to deal with them.

3. The *Blue plans* (Blue Cross for hospital costs, Blue Shield for physician charges) were created in the Depression years by hospitals and physicians, in response to such widespread inability of the public to meet medical bills that payment of a discounted bill seemed a vast improvement over no payment at all. It can plausibly be argued that these volunteer community efforts prevented the collapse of the private medical system or the creation of a government-run health system of the Scandinavian or British variety. (Lacking a vigorous voluntary insurance system, Canada did move much further toward a government-run system, and the transition to the present Canadian national health insurance system was considerably advanced by the steps taken by the Canadian government during the Great Depression.) Most of the problems now posed by the Blue plans grew out of failure to modify the premises which were appropriate to the 1930's. Payment on a discounted basis, rather than full payment, persists as a principle in both Blue Cross and Blue Shield; retrospective cost-reimbursement remains the predominant method of Blue Cross payment

(instead of paying the itemized charges which others must pay), and their non-profit corporate structures have persisted even though the larger plans approach a billion dollars in annual turnover. Blue plans usually escape premium taxes which are typically 2 percent, and this advantage plus the existence of contractual discounts from hospitals has allowed aggressive plans to become virtual health insurance monopolies in some areas like the East coast. If the hospitals and physicians who initially provided the seed capital, discounts and management had been less selfless in forming non-profit corporations, the Blue plans would have sold shares to stockholders and there might now be less competitive advantage. Instead, states are increasingly prodded by the Federal Trade Commission to pass laws forbidding hospitals and doctors to sit on the boards of directors of corporations they founded. It might be much wiser to limit the market share of non-profit health insurance companies, since a regulated monopoly with a "public" board is a very short step from a government agency. Only the present tax hunger of both state and federal governments exists as an incentive for governments to turn back from the trend toward government ownership of the health insurance industry.[2]

Blue plan share of the entire market even in the East was considerably diminished by the advent of Medicare, which took away a large number of subscribers with a heavy illness experience. On the other hand, Medicare and Medicaid copied the Blue Cross system of retrospective cost-reimbursement. Since the government merely supervises Medicare and Medicaid and the actual administration is conducted by contract with private organizations acting as intermediaries,[3] it was fairly natural for the great majority of these lucrative contracts to go to Blue plans. Since the non-profit corporations never had profitability at risk, it has made very little

2. An interesting twist exists in the 1979 Kennedy proposal for National Health Insurance. While both the Carter and the Kennedy proposals include a role for the private health insurance companies, the Kennedy proposal envisions a graduated payroll tax which would be fed into a pool of funds to pay premiums. The premiums would be "community rated" which means that the taxation would be proportional to income rather than sickness probability. While the insurance industry at first was pleased to be included, they began to draw back as they considered how foreign this approach would be to their present operation, and how close it would be to nationalization of the health insurance industry. Public boards of directors, appointed by regulatory rules and excluding providers of care, would presumably be much less resistant to the concept of progressive taxation.

3. For some reason, the companies acting as administrators for Medicare Part B are called "carriers."

difference to Blue plan intermediaries whether the business was governmental or their own. The effect was largely one of expanding the previous activity. It would be going too far to say that America already has National Health Insurance (NHI) in the Blue Cross-government combination. But it is certainly no exaggeration that the nonprofit health insurance industry fully expects to be the vehicle for any NHI of the future, and that it does not expect serious inconvenience from the change.[4]

4. The *commercial health insurance* industry is made up of over three hundred companies, and it is accordingly difficult to describe briefly. Some companies are owned by stockholders, some owned by the policy holders (mutuals), some (like Lloyd's of London) have the underwriter at total personal risk for losses. Some companies are large, many are small. Some solicit business by direct mail, some work only with groups of subscribers. Some act only as reinsurers of risk, some are largely a shell for reinsurance companies. One of the most important new trends, to be described in Chapter 14, is not to insure at all, but to act as an administrator for self-insured groups.

The normal method of operation for commercial carriers of health insurance is about as follows:

A. INDEMNITY (i.e., dollar) benefits instead of "Service Benefits." Service benefits (i.e., we pay for your sickness no matter what it costs) are much more characteristic of the Blue plans, and force them into wrangling with the hospitals about prices and costs, for which purpose they need a contract signed by the hospital. The commercial carriers normally avoid this issue by offering to pay a fixed sum per day in hospital, leaving the subscriber liable to pay any balance of the charges.

B. NO CONTRACT WITH THE HOSPITAL. The commercial insurer has a contract with the subscriber to reimburse the subscriber for certain stated expenses, but is under no obligation to deal directly with the hospitals. Paradoxically, payments made to hospitals for services rendered commercial subscribers are sometimes more prompt than Blue plan payments. Most patients execute an assignment of benefits form at the time of admission to hospital, and the claim processing departments of the commercial carriers some-

4. In Canada, the Blue plans did act as intermediaries for the Canadian National Health Scheme, but the relationship lasted only a short time.

times can outperform the direct relationship with hospitals established by Blue plan hospital contracts. Unfortunately, the high
interest rates of recent inflationary times have encouraged all
payers to slow down their payable systems to take advantage of
interest on the money. Hospitals are just as guilty in their transactions with their suppliers as health insurance companies are with
hospitals, and it is difficult to know how the cycle is to stop. The
payable freeze does tend to obscure the claims efficiency of the
other companies. Therefore, efficient companies are the last to
begin and the first to discontinue the practice of deliberate slow
pay whenever the business cycle heats up.

C. AGE-STRATIFIED PREMIUMS. Since sickness costs get larger as
you get older there is an obvious subsidy created when the
premium is uniform no matter how old the employee is. Thus,
indemnity companies can make an attractive offer to young groups.

5. *Self-pay*. Having described briefly the major kinds of situations involving insurance, we are now ready to discuss the plight of
a fifth group, the patients who have no hospital insurance at all. A
typical person each year has about one chance in seven of being
admitted to a hospital, and thus developing a bill of about two
thousand dollars. Since young people are healthier and run up
smaller bills when they do get sick, the risk for a person age 30
might be guessed to be less than 200 dollars a year. A person age 55
may well be running the risk of $500 dollars a year, but he has had
more years in the labor force to accumulate savings for this
purpose. Such risks, while not inconsequential, are mostly bearable. Since typical health insurance premiums are appreciably
higher than these estimates, it is apparent that the benefit packages
have been extended beyond the major financial hazard of hospitalization into more routine costs in the outpatient area. This burden-
ing of the premium grew out of a plausible well-intentioned theory.
It was reasoned that patients might be unnecessarily admitted to
hospitals in order to have their hospitalization insurance cover
services which could have been performed more cheaply on an
outpatient basis. Hence, the theory ran, the benefits should be
extended to cover such outpatient services, with a resulting decrease in the overall cost. This theory has gained wide currency,
and whatever its merits, has markedly increased the scope of
health insurance. Its merits are probably small, and its secondary

consequences outweigh them. For example, it is not unusual for claims processing costs to range around six dollars a claim. Clearly there are some unfortunate consequences from a theory which invokes the insurance mechanism for a three dollar urinalysis. It should be fairly easy to examine the before-and-after experience in localities which switched to the inclusion of outpatient benefits in the hospitalization package, and it will then be possible to judge whether significant abuse existed in health plans which failed to provide outpatient coverage. No doubt there was some abuse. The important question is whether extending insurance coverage to small outpatient items caused a greater administrative cost than the in-patient abuse it was intended to abate.

The issue is sometimes raised whether young Americans of average income might find it prudent to "go bare" of health insurance. For example, young subscribers are obviously subsidizing older subscribers when the premium makes no allowance for the age of the client. In view of the fact that pregnancy is a condition which can (for the most part) be planned for, the heaviest portion of even the age-rated premium for young people may not be an item which is sensibly included in an insurance package. After all, a sound insurable risk is one which cannot be anticipated, and one which is considered by the insured to be a disaster which he hopes to avoid. There is room to argue that young persons should budget their pregnancies, and that other financial health risks are too remote to worry about. Go bare, in other words, but be careful of pregnancy.

At the other end of the spectrum, there are many older persons who have enjoyed years of health and prosperity, and who have accumulated, say five or ten thousand dollars in reserves. Their need is for catastrophic coverage, not routine health insurance, and their reserves would cover all but 1 percent of hospitalizations for persons under Medicare age. It is true that this age group can now obtain health insurance at unrealistically low premiums through the subsidy from younger subscribers. But even so, why not spend premium money on a vacation?

The answer is don't do it, on the basis entirely of dollars and cents rather than of protection. Reduced to its crudest form, it can be said that one reason to buy certain forms of health insurance is that your employer is paying for it, and there is an income tax subsidy to keep him doing so. A second reason is to avoid being overcharged anywhere up to 35 percent.

Take an example: If half of a hospital's patients receive a 5 percent discount, the remaining half must pay a 5 percent premium, and there is a 10 percent difference in what the two groups pay. But much more, if 90 percent of the patients received a 5 percent discount, the remaining 10 percent of the patients must pay a 45 percent premium to balance the books, and there is a 50 percent difference in what the two groups pay for the same service. This "Blue Cross discount" varies in amount in different areas at different times; it is not restricted to Blue Cross plans (Medicare and Medical Assistance cases also participate); in some areas of the country the analysis does not pertain at all; and it is true that overcharging the other patients is a voluntary act of the hospital and not specifically mandated by contract. Since the cost payers by reason of contract do not pay this "discount," it is referred to by the term "contractual allowance." Surprisingly few people know it exists but the contractual allowance is one of the most potent forces at work in the health system.[5]

Various qualifiers on the discount (or contractual allowance) situation are:

1.   Usually the discount disappears when hospitals participate in a "negotiated *charge*" type of contract rather than on a "negotiated *cost*" basis. The discount in a *cost* negotiation grows out of lengthy arguments about "allowable" costs. The same arguments can take place, item by item, in a negotiated *charge* contract, where they can be lumped into a residual daily charge which is very loosely called a room and board charge. However, it remains generally true that there is more uniformity of charges in various patient charge classes in Blue Cross plan areas which employ a negotiated charge system.

2.   The arithmetic given in the examples illustrates that the gearing of the cost differential would be greatest in those regions with the highest market penetration by the cost reimbursement third parties. At some point, the difference between "cost" and "charges" becomes so great that competitors are driven out, and the question of monopoly abuse has to be seriously asked.

5. A Chicago Hospital Council study recently showed that patients in that area who pay their own bills are forced to pay $23 per day extra ($191 per hospitalization) to cover underpayments by Medicare and Medicaid. Blue Cross was not mentioned.

3. The Medicare program was modelled on the Blue Cross system, and mostly uses Blue Cross employees on an administrative contract. Medical Assistance has certain differences, but it too can be lumped with Blue Cross and Medicare as a "cost reimburser." Therefore the gearing of the cost discount suddenly became unbearable after the sudden introduction of the two government programs; but the likelihood of a successful antitrust suit was comparably diminished. As a sidelight on the issue, it seems to be true that Medicare is somewhat overcharged by comparison with Blue Cross and Medical Assistance. True costs are much higher in the first few days of hospitalization. Since Medicare pays its share of a flat daily room cost, and since the elderly stay on in the hospital several days longer than average, with a level per diem rate, any such group with long average length of stay gets overcharged.

4. In an ordinary for-profit corporation there is a tension between customers who want low prices, and stockholders who want high profits. Since Blue plans lack the profit motive, the pressure on management is almost entirely in the direction of lowering the premiums to the customers. The pressure is all the more tenacious when the customers begin to people the board of directors with union officers and corporate personnel managers. Indeed, Adam Smith would weep to contemplate the utter impossibility of selecting "public" board members who had no bias toward using market power to maintain Blue Cross market share, and, hence, subsidy to themselves.

5. Since the discount partly grows out of accounting arguments over "allowable" costs, it should be recognized that some hospital costs really might not be allowable. Opulent administrative quarters, excessive salaries, overstaffing, unnecessary equipment and capacity might conceivably develop without some outside review. Or, unfunded capital depreciation and unfunded pensions might distort the balance sheet.

Such delicate matters as these are seldom the contemporary basis for disagreement. The two issues, which are not without merit on both sides, are:
• Charity and its blurred extension, bad debts.
• A margin of safety, or operating margin for contingencies and invisible attrition of assets.
The cost reimbursement auditors see no reason why they should

pay for credit risks when their patients present no credit risk. An extension of this argument is that they should not pay for charity care when they have made the contribution of removing many of their subscribers from the charity rolls. Furthermore, "margin of safety" is too nebulous a term for an auditor; if you can't define it, you can't justify it. And as for the hardship we impose on the clients of our competitors, well, business is business.

7

A Primer from the Trustees

Mr. Stokes and Mr. Wynne walked briskly down the hospital corridor to the administration office. Waiting for them was a third man, well-dressed. All shook hands, and greeted each other warmly.

"Hi, Tim," said the courtly Mr. Wynne. "This is your first meeting of the budget and finance committee, isn't it? Bill Stokes and I have been coming to these sessions for too many years. Now we can hope to be able to share the headaches with some young eager fellows."

All three smiled at the pleasantry since Mr. Matlack, the newcomer, was clearly a few years older than the others. But he was their junior in service on the Board of Trustees, and good-humored about his need for instruction. The three entered the administrative workroom where they found the chairman of the committee, Mr. Scattergood, already seated at the table, Mr. Scattergood, who looked like a Roman senator, was a successful bank president, scrupulous always to be a few minutes early for any appointment. It was one of many characteristics of a person that everybody liked and wanted to do things for. A gentle man, he almost never raised his voice and had reached his position in life by persuasion and fairness. A nice guy, and no dummy.

The four members of the finance committee were immediately joined by the comptroller of the hospital, Oscar O'Toole. The room buzzed with courteous amiability as these men of affairs promptly arranged themselves for business. Without officiousness, Mr. Scattergood invited the comptroller to begin the meeting, and Mr. O'Toole said: "You gentlemen will be as thrilled as I was to discover that next year the hospital's budget is going to be almost exactly one hundred million. When I arrived fifteen years ago I never dreamed the budget would reach that size."

There were appreciative murmurs and raised eyebrows as the members of the committee, accustomed to large numbers, had to admit that one hundred million dollars was real money. Mr. Stokes smiled and said, "At least round numbers like that will make it easier to follow your presentation, Oscar. Personally, I was always slow at math."

Mr. Scattergood looked up. "In the forty years your father was on the board of this hospital, Bill, there were probably fewer changes than we have seen in the last two or three years. Mr. O'Toole, of the hundred-million-dollar budget, how much do you actually expect we will have to spend?"

"Oh," said Mr. O'Toole, "all of it. The hundred million represents actual projected expenditures for the year."

"My goodness. How large do you project the necessary revenue to be?"

"Well," said Mr. O'Toole, "perhaps just a little more, for safety. Perhaps an extra half million as a cushion."

"Maybe I'm a pessimist," said Mr. Stokes, "but I just don't feel comfortable in my business without a 3 percent cushion. Too many things go wrong that you darned well can't predict. We might have a strike, or one of our prize surgeons might take a long well-earned vacation in Brazil."

"Yea, verily," said Mr. Wynne, "in these inflationary times, I would think even 3 percent is a dangerously narrow margin. Just think, if inflation should go up 13 percent this year, as God help us some people are predicting, you could soak up an average of 6 or 7 percent right there."

"Yes, I think you are all correct," said Mr. Scattergood. "Shall we set the revenue goal at one hundred five million? It's a frightening number, but I think we would be irresponsible not to face facts. We can't be precise in our advance estimates, so we have to aim a little high at the beginning of the year. Are we agreed?"

"Please," said the newcoming Timothy Matlack, "I'm not sure what you're talking about. If we need a hundred million, why are we trying to get a hundred and five?"

"Tim, we don't know what we'll actually get. Right now, we're talking about setting a level of charges for the services the hospital renders. We have to guess how much money a certain set of charges will generate.

"It's our job on the finance committee to set a revenue goal, and then Mr. O'Toole here will tinker with the individual charges to try to achieve that goal. He'll charge ten dollars for this and a thousand dollars for that, but it's all supposed to aim for the revenue goal we set. Or rather, that the Board of Trustees will set at their next meeting when they get the recommendation of this committee. As the year goes along, Oscar may be able to see that his charges aren't meeting the goal month by month, so he may have to readjust the charge schedule several times. But the sum total is supposed to hit the goal we set."

"Why not set it for a hundred million, and adjust for that? Isn't that what you want to achieve in a nonprofit institution?"

"Look, Tim, let's take a longer view of the institution. If you ever end up a year with less than your costs, you have no choice but to overcharge next year's patients for the fact that this year's patients didn't pay their own way. We've had plenty of years when we had to do that, and it doesn't give you a good feeling, believe me. So you aim a little high. Sometimes you come out high, sometimes right on the nose, and sometimes you come out low in spite of aiming high. Now, there's another thing to consider.

"In spite of the talents of our fine financial staff, there is always some undefinable attrition. That's particularly true in an institution that receives gifts and bequests. Certain assets are invisibly used up, and you must make provision for replacing them. There are also improvements which become necessary as the year goes along, and you need to have a cushion so management doesn't have to come to the board for authorization every time there is a decision to switch from quill pens to ballpoints.

"Now, this sort of need, plus the uncertainty of precisely reaching your goal, means that there is a cushion which experience shows you better have. Over the years, this institution has found that 5 percent advance projected margin comes pretty close to bringing us out right, even though it may take several years for the hills and valleys to smooth out. The whole thing is more of an art than a science, it differs between hospitals, and therefore it properly is a board responsibility to set the figure. Over the long haul, the institution prospers or shrivels depending on how well we make our guess." Mr. Matlack listened in silence, and nodded approval.

Mr. O'Toole entered the discussion. "The size of the advance projected surplus is one of the major reasons the contractual allowances are so high."

At this, Mr. Matlack, who had been tipping his chair backward, set it forward with a clatter. "I guess it's time for me to admit something. I really don't understand what contractual allowances are all about. I've been reading them in annual reports for the last three years. They look like a huge amount of lost revenue, and I think it's an outrage that we permit these third parties to gouge us that way. What's the matter with us that we let them get away with it? Why don't we go out in the community and stir up the issue so that a stop is put to it? After all, it's our government, and once in a while it can be persuaded to do the sensible thing."

Mr. Scattergood twinkled. "I'm so glad you asked. Nothing is quite so misunderstood, and you might even say misrepresented. But if you expect to serve on this committee and still keep your sanity, you'll have to understand it. Mr. O'Toole, give it to him straight. Talk slowly, and use the flip chart over there."

Mr. O'Toole walked over to the blank paper on a tripod, and picked up a green felt marking pen. "In our hospital, the composition of patients is as follows:

"Cost" Reimbursed	80%
Charge "Reimbursed"	20
	100%

"I put quotation marks around 'cost' and the second 'reimbursement,' because the 'cost' they reimburse is determined by formulas which I don't happen to agree with. And the charges they 'reimburse' include all of our charity work and dead beats."

Mr. Matlack showed interest. "How much is charity?"

"About two million dollars worth."

"Two percent."

"Right."

"OK, how does the cost-reimbursement split up among Blue Cross, Medicare, and Medical Assistance?"

"In our hospital," replied O'Toole, "it would be as follows:

COST REIMBURSED	
Medicare	40%
Medical Assistance	20
Blue Cross	20
	80%.

"Now to go on. The cost-reimbursed patients are paid for on the basis of audited costs, no matter what charges they run up. The other 20 percent of patients pay the charges, no matter what the costs may have been. So the only purpose of setting charges is to determine how much revenue we will obtain from that 20 percent. It's true that we send a bill to each of the other patients, but it's marked paid in full, and what it says on the bill really has nothing to do with what we are actually paid later by Medicare, Medicaid, and Blue Cross. Because we agree to this in a contract, it is called a contractual allowance.

"Now, as a matter of fact, Medicare, Medicaid, and Blue Cross don't even pay all of their costs. They send their team of auditors and say 'This isn't allowed, that isn't an allowable cost, we can't agree to something else!' "

Mr. Matlack thought he was following. "So what they cut out and refuse to pay for is the contractual allowance, and it was eighteen million dollars last year?"

"No, no," said Mr. O'Toole, "that isn't the contractual allowance at all. Those are the disallowed costs."

"How much?"

"About two percent."

"About two million. But last year the contractual allowances were listed as eighteen million, and I was mad as the devil at Blue Cross."

"Okay," said O'Toole, "let me show you." He went to the flip chart and wrote:

Advance Projected Surplus	$5,000,000
Disallowed Costs	2,000,000
Total "Crunch"	$7,000,000

"The 'crunch' is made up of the two main ingredients we have talked about. The crunch is the amount of money we have to have, and 80 percent of our patients don't contribute a dime toward it."

"Go ahead," said Matlack.

"And so we have to get that money from the 20 percent of our patients who pay their charges as follows:

Fair Proportion of Costs	$20,000,000 (100%)
Crunch	7,000,000 (33)
Total Charges to Charge Payers	$27,000,000 (133%)

Matlack reddened. "That's unbelievable."

Mr. Scattergood smiled. "Other people have had stronger words for it."

"But wait a minute. The figures make it look as though Blue Cross, Medicare, and Medicaid get a 33 percent discount, but they don't at all. They are getting a 2 percent discount, or maybe a 7 percent discount if you want to argue that point about operating margin."

"Oh, we do argue it. Every year at audit time."

"All right, you've educated me, but if I understand contractual allowances, I've just forgotten why I understand them. Last year you wrote in the annual report that we lost eighteen million through contractual allowances. That's how much the cost reimbursement agencies should have paid and didn't, right?"

"Right"

"Well, why is it only two million, or seven million, this year?"

"It isn't. It's thirty-six million. Let me show you:

COST-REIMBURSED PATIENTS (80%)		CHARGE-REIMBURSED PATIENTS (20%)
Costs (basic)	$ 80,000,000	$20,000,000
Costs (basic & 5%)	84,000,000	21,000,000
Payments	78,400,000	26,600,000
Charges	115,080,000	28,600,000
Contractual Allowance:	$ 36,680,000 Charity:	$ 2,000,000
(CHARITY AND UNREIMBURSED DISCOUNTS		$38,680,000)

REVENUES		
Beyond Costs (basic & 5%)		$ 5,600,000
Beyond Costs (basic)		6,600,000
Below Costs (basic & 5%)	5,600,000	
Below Costs (basic)	1,600,000	

Mr. Matlack walked to the flip chart, "But you are displaying those charges as if they were the fair-market price in a profit-making business, when in fact they are just padding for the books. You are living on an expense account.

Now it's true that you are on an expense account that only pays 98 cents on the dollar, but that doesn't give you any right to claim that you were cheated out of 36 cents profit. As I see it, the fair way to display the situation is as follows:

COST REIMBURSED PATIENTS (80%)		CHARGE REIMBURSED PATIENTS (20%)
Costs	$80,000,000	$20,000,000
Payments	79,000,000	27,000,000
	($ 1,000,000)	$ 7,000,000

"By rounding off, the numbers don't quite come out in balance, but you see what I mean. The contractual allowance is an accountant's fiction. If our charge-paying patients should only represent 5 percent of the clients instead of 20 percent, you could fiddle around with the figures until the contractual allowances would be $130 million. Implying you lost $130 million with expenses of only $100 million. Now look, even the federal government would have trouble losing more money per year than it spends per year.

COST REIMBURSED PATIENTS (95%)		CHARGE REIMBURSED PATIENTS (5%)
Charges	$223,000,000	$12,000,000
Payments	93,000,000	12,000,000
Contractual Allowance	$130,000,000	0
(COSTS $100,000,000, REVENUES $105,000,000)		

"It seems to me," said Matlack, getting warmer, "that things are outrageous enough without trying to score points with magic. Your only hope of rescue is that the public can be brought to understand this mess, and you just make it tougher for yourself with razzle-dazzle. The cost-reimbursed third-party payment agencies owe us two million bucks, or seven million at the most. Period. You aren't going to make any friends by trying to represent it as thirty-six million."

Mr. Scattergood silently invited Mr. Matlack to calm down, with an amused look. "It certainly is true that no strong case is improved by exaggeration, Tim. Perhaps we could ask Oscar here to recast the annual report to the contributors so that it reflects our affairs along the lines Mr. Matlack is suggesting." Mr. O'Toole looked troubled and started to object, but stopped himself before he uttered a word. Mr. Scattergood noticed.

"You know," Scattergood decided to continue, "Joe and I have some friends over in Maryland who are on the boards of some of the hospitals. They got themselves worked up into a lather a few years ago about the contractual allowances, and went to the Maryland legislature about it. Uniform reimbursement was the battlecry. As you might imagine, the local Blue Cross lobbied hard against it, and there was a lot of bad feeling. Well, they ended up with a new level of bureaucracy to fight with, called something like the State of Maryland Hospital Rate Commission. And since the federal programs wouldn't go along with it, they still have contractual allowances in Maryland. I really would be fearful to get our loyal contributors, patients, and friends all stirred up about something they don't understand very well. The outcome might well be a situation which is worse."

Mr. Stokes leaned back in his chair as a way of asking for a turn to speak, and the group turned toward him. "One of the sort of frightening things about contractual allowances is the way the Bureau of Labor Statistics includes them in the health component of the cost of living index."

"I wasn't aware of that," answered Mr. Wynne. "How did you find that out?"

"It's no secret. One of the people from my place was down in Washington talking to them on another matter. As a matter of fact, he suggested they use the Medicare cost reports which go to the Social Security Administration, but that's only filed once a year. The Labor Department feels it needs monthly figures for the cost of living index, so it uses patient charges instead of true costs."

"Typical bureaucracy," said Mr. Stokes. "They think it's better to use the wrong numbers every month than the right numbers once a year."

Mr. Wynne turned to Mr. Matlack. "So you see, Tim, from the Bureau of Labor Statistics' point of view, our next year's budget is one hundred forty-three million. That's the hundred million that O'Toole brought in here, plus the five million we added, plus thirty-six million more of phoney baloney that we call contractual allowances."

"Wow," said Matlack.

"Do you have any further comments for the record, Mr. Matlack?" asked Mr. Scattergood.

"No," said Matlack, "Wow says it all."

"In that case, I guess the meeting is over for this month. Can I give anyone a ride to the station? We'll just leave Mr. O'Toole here with the wreckage. His big job now is to sharpen up his pencil and see how much of that seven million he can get back for us. I don't know how he manages to do it, but almost every year somehow those losses mostly get cut down to size."

8

Further Subsidies

The late Dr. Richard Chamberlain, who at that time was chairman of the X-ray department in a large teaching hospital, described his department's charging policy as follows: "I can prove that it actually costs $1,700 to perform a coronary arteriogram, but we only charge $250; we make it up by charging $35 for a whole lot of $5 chest X-rays." Few radiologists would dispute that many other charges are also disconnected from actual costs. Neither would most pathologists deny that many of the innovative and expensive procedures in their departments are subsidized by the routine work. Nor bacteriologists, nor anaesthesiologists. And most of them would say that such pricing distortions are traditional for reasons that are obscure to them. So let us explore the rationality of the pricing system, and allow the reader to decide what he thinks of it.

We have seen that hospital revenues come from two quite distinct sources. One group (Blue Cross, Medicare, and Medicaid) pays costs, the other group (commercial indemnity insurance, cash paying uninsureds, and uninsured bad debts) pays charges (cost plus profit). It is to the hospital's advantage if the cost-reimbursement group pays maximum costs, and the charge-reimbursement group pays maximum charges. It's almost that simple. Costs and charges have little to do with each other, so the result is a bizarre and irregular ratio of costs to charges (also known as a mark-up, or profit margin).

Let us first examine the perspective of the cost accountant. For reasons that are immaterial to him and this discussion, the various services and departments of the hospital are quite nonuniform in their usage by the two payment systems. Some departments are used almost exclusively by cost-reimbursed patients, others (like the emergency room) concentrate the bad debts, still others are used by outpatients. We will return to outpatients, but at this point it is important to notice that Medicare will reimburse 100 percent of inpatient costs, but only 80 percent of outpatient costs. The obstetrical delivery room is used exclusively by inpatients, but the electrocardiographic department may do substantial ambulatory work. The obvious strategy is to assign as many costs as possible to the labor room and as few costs as possible to the emergency room. But how to do this?

Costs are forcibly divided into "direct" costs and "indirect" costs through a theory which states that every cost must be assigned to a payment.[1] Take the matter of mowing the lawn, for example. It costs money to cut the grass, but no patient gets a bill for grass. Grass cutting is an indirect cost of running the whole institution. It is admittedly a pretty arbitrary matter how grass-cutting, telephone operating, general administration, and a multitude of other matters are assigned to particular patient bills. The hazy qualities of indirect costs are very suitable. If no one really knows where to put them, it is legitimate to put them into departments which mostly reimburse costs. A shrewd cost accountant will avoid putting them in departments that have bad debts. Given a choice, avoid assigning them to departments with a large amount of ambulatory work.

Since indirect costs can be shifted around to a certain degree, it is important to take every opportunity to place a cost in the indirect category if that can be managed. An example might be the security guard or the nursing supervisor for the emergency room. If assigned to that area, their salaries become direct costs of the emergency room. But placed in a general pool of security guards or nursing supervision for the whole hospital, they become indirect costs. It is generally found that about 50 to 70 percent of current hospital costs can be placed in the indirect category.

One should not suppose that the assignment of indirect costs to individual "charge centers" is entirely without constraint. An

---

1. The purpose of this theory is to achieve a way of employing charges to determine a fair proportion of costs for each payer class. See Chapter 9, "Fair Shares."

auditable theory must be followed. For example, grass cutting might be assigned to departments on the basis of the number of employees in the department (theory: more people trample more grass). Or security guard costs might be assigned proportionate to departmental payroll (theory: more money to steal). Or, to be less frivolous, the housekeeping, heating, air conditioning, and building maintenance might be assigned on the basis of the number of square feet of floor space in the department.

There are two serious flaws in this system. The first is the fairly obvious fact that some high-use areas of the hospital require a disproportionately larger housekeeping and painting maintenance, quite unrelated to their floor space. The darker second problem is the temptation which is created to enlarge the floor space of a cost-reimbursed department, and constrain the floor area of a charge-reimbursed department. When responses of this sort are stimulated, the process changes from cost-shifting to cost escalation.

We have now gone through the main outline of the process whereby costs are assigned to categories (if in doubt, call it an indirect cost), and indirect costs are sprinkled among the reimbursement centers (assign as much as possible to departments where costs reimbursement is highest). One significant variation on the cost reimbursement side is the nursing care cost differential, and one major abstraction is the subject of borrowing and depreciation. These last two issues are so important that they are treated separately elsewhere.

The first step in the process is complete. All of the hospital costs which, with any excuse, can be shifted to the cost-reimbursement agencies ("the Feds") have been shifted. Let the uninsured patient and the commercial indemnity insurance companies take note. There is no choice but to dump the rest of the costs on the small group of patients who have no contract with the hospital, therefore having no right to a contractual "allowance." They have to pay the full charges, and the charges must be raised high enough to break even.

Turning now to that small group of defenseless payers, who have been sheltered so far as ingenuity can devise, we now see that the survival of the hospital depends on their paying for whatever residual costs remain. We also see that it makes no difference to them what things really cost, or even what things are fancied to cost, if the patient pays charges. The issue is only that he pays the charge. Thus, a distinction must be imagined between the charges which will be reimbursed no matter how high they are (example: covered by a major medical commercial policy) and the charges which may evaporate into bad debts if they get too expensive. There is also the restraint that excessive charges in the ambulatory area may be undercut by outside commercial laboratories responding to the competitive challenge. Because the hospital may have to restrain itself on ambulatory or emergency room charges, it exaggerates charges which major medical plans would cover. Transfusions and intensive care units get charges which are particularly extreme.

We are not quite through with the ratio of costs to charges. The hospital financial manager might wish that the two were totally unrelated, since it would free him to put charges as high as the market will bear. That is the system used in pricing computers on what IBM calls a "value-related" rather than a cost-related basis. However, it is not so simple. The cost-reimbursement agencies calculate their share of a department's activity on the basis of their client's proportion of charges. That is, charges have nothing to do with costs, but apportionment of costs has something to do with charges. We have looked at the first cycle of cost apportionment; there are later cycles. The process of raising chest X-ray charges to cash customers may have the undesired effect of drawing some of the cost apportionment away from the cost reimbursers, since their fair share is determined by the porportion of charges incurred by their clients. There probably is a profitable business opportunity for a computer soft-ware company to design a modeling program which would optimize the hospital charging system. Lacking this, the present problem in understanding and explaining hospital charge policy is that, to a certain degree, it is fully understood by no one at all, since secondary cross-relationships shift the original premises. Thus, a department which is mostly used by cost reimbursers may cease to be maximally reimbursed by those who pay the cost if the wrong charges are raised. The whole system is called "charges proportional to charges, applied to costs.[2]"

2. See Chapter 9, "Fair Shares."

OVERVIEW

No discussion of hospital reimbursement practices is complete without describing distortions caused by the nursing care cost differential, the failure to collect coinsurance, nonreplacement fees for Red Cross blood donations, and the chronic renal dialysis program. But these inflammatory subjects distract from understanding the central process. It is hoped that a brief overview of the main elements is sufficient to permit a preliminary judgment of the system's effect on fundamentals. What should we think about all this?

The aphorism which seems to fit best is Arnold Toynbee's conclusion about the rise and fall of civilizations: Human organizations often destroy themselves by overextending their best features. The modern American hospital is the envy of the world for its quality of care, its research, its teaching, its charity, and its high level of amenity. The reimbursement system made it all possible; any change in the reimbursement system may destroy it all. But failure to examine the reimbursement system critically will also destroy it all.

It should first be noticed that the dual nature of the reimbursement sources is basic to both the distortions of the present system and to its survival. There are a few hospitals which have no private or commercial reimbursement sources, but they are rapidly being driven to the wall. Philadelphia General Hospital, until five years ago the largest hospital in the State of Pennsylvania, has been closed. The City of New York is proposing to close half of its municipal hospital system, totaling tens of thousands of beds. The story is being repeated across the country, so that hospitals which trained the bulk of nurses and house officers for two centuries may be doomed. One city administration after another is discovering that retrospective cost-reimbursement never covers every need, that standard bureaucratic responses like fixed prospective budgets, deferred maintenance, and job freezes will not mitigate auditor-enforced retrospective denials, and that eventually you go broke. Retrospective cost reimbursement of hospitals cannot be tolerated unless at least some self-pay and commercially insured patients are forced to pay a markup, to cover the cost-reimbursement exclusions. It is this small vital part of the system which is now breaking down, and the breakdown occurs first in those hospitals which have the smallest proportion of patients paying full charges.

The markup (between "costs" and charges) is now about 35 percent in Philadelphia hospitals. The size of the markup is determined by the proportion of patients available to pay it. For many years, the unpaid contractual allowance or "Blue Cross discount" was 5 to 7 percent. While that was hard to justify, it did not drive out commercial competition in most areas of the country. However, when Medicare and Medicaid (1965-66) adopted the cost reimbursement system, suddenly the great majority of patients were reimbursed at "cost." Whenever the proportion of patients paying posted charges shrank to 10 to 15 percent, the markup had to be raised to 30 percent, or even more disheartening levels. Commercial insurance companies could not compete, so commercial health insurance tends to become almost unobtainable except through large employee groups (and usually only groups known to be predominatly young and healthy).

The higher the markup, the harder it becomes to get commercial insurance; but it is also true that the less commercial indemnity insurance, the higher the markup. At some point in such a spiral, payment of charges will disappear entirely, with the affected hospitals placed in the position of Cook County Hospital and Philadelphia General Hospital. Since the country obviously will not tolerate the destruction of its hospitals (once it is convinced by some spectacular examples), the chilling prospect appears that continuation of the present spiral may lead to regulatory or legislative solutions of the Canadian and British sort (see Chapter 19).

THE NEW CHARITY MECHANISM

That the road to hospital perdition is paved with good intentions is illustrated in several ways. For an example we might look at the 6 percent of Americans totally outside the insurance-and-welfare system who, in addition to the patients whose illnesses exceed their insurance coverage, constitute the major source of bad debts for hospitals. The bad debt is, as we have seen, inflated 35 percent by the markup over "costs," but 50 to 70 percent of these costs are of the indirect variety and hence often understated if the accountant is skillful. Apparent losses (charges) are exaggerated, and real losses (costs) are minimized. It is true that the hospital's best interest is parallel to the best interest of the uninsured semi-indigent patient, but it is ungracious to snipe at motivation. The system does have some social merit.

In this bizarre and arcane way, the traditional Robin Hood system is still vigorous in hospitals, although now the insurance mechanism rather than the prewar "private" patient plays the involuntary role of fat burger of Nottingham. The commercial insurance companies are perhaps disproportionately victimized by the process, but Blue Cross, Medicare, and Medicaid do not escape. Indirect costs are shifted around so that "cost" reimbursement subsidizes charge reimbursement, and what's more, the premiums of Blue Cross group subscribers are inflated to subsidize the nongroup Blue Cross subscriber.[3] It can fairly be argued that nongroup Blue Cross subscribers would greatly increase the number of hospital bad debts if they could not obtain their subsidized coverage. The issue is so complex that it is hard to be sure just where the balance lies between the commercial carriers and their nonprofit competitor. In view of the near monopoly by Blue Cross in some areas, however, external circumstances suggest that Blue Cross receives somewhat lighter treatment.

So all of the Byzantine complexity of the hospital accounting system may well be forgivable for the fact that it does tend to reduce the cost of hospitalization for the uninsured group who now can least afford hospitalization. After all, the first step in the cost accounting treatment is to shift as many costs as possible on to the cost-reimbursed, service-benefit patients. But, having first done what he can to shelter the uninsured or out-of-benefits patient, there is no doubt the hospital accountant then lays the rest of it on the back of the charge-reimbursed group. It's them or us.

We are not through with the point, however. At the same time that the insurance mechanism is being internally extended to subsidize the uninsured somewhat, hospital costs are thereby further released from the restraint that no one can afford them. There would be no need for insurance if hospital costs were trivial. By promoting extravagance, insurance makes itself more essential, and moral hazard ensnares insurance companies and welfare

3. It is usually the insurance commissioner who forces this subsidy.

bureaucracies. We are now at the point in public perception where it is recognized, by students of the matter at least, that medical costs have gone up too rapidly for the principal reason that there is a moral hazard.[4] Most people also dimly recognize that there is probably something wrong with extending mandatory insurance to the last 6 percent who do not have it, if pervasiveness of insurance moral hazard was the basic problem in the first place. The dilemma of the cost accountant is that his techniques both mitigate pain for the uninsured, and cause pain to be made worse for society.

PAYING FOR SCIENTIFIC INNOVATION

So much for charity; let us look at innovation. The system we are describing has been extremely successful in promoting scientific innovation. A glance at England or Canada provides a pointed contrast. Innovation should be distinguished from research, and is intended to mean the development and dissemination of new techniques and technology. It is here that Dr. Chamberlain's charging algorithm begins to make some sense. Insurance companies have a tendency to resist charges for things they never heard of; new procedures are now generally held down until the procedure has proven itself. Therefore, prices on established procedures are kited to pay for new and partly untried ones. The cost reimbursement agencies especially subsidize innovative procedures for the uninsured.

Unfortunately, this process grossly deceives the attending physician as to what things cost. A physician who conscientiously attempts to consider the relative costs of various management strategies may well be encouraged to order more coronary arteriograms and to hold back on chest X-rays. To the extent that costly procedures might supplant cheap ones, the system is being pushed in exactly the wrong direction.

Distortion of medical care by cross subsidies is not limited to technology. Since the daily room charge is exclusively an inpatient cost (at 100 percent reimbursement) while most laboratory and

4. The tendency for individuals to incur more expenses when these expenses are insured than when they are not is often referred to as the "moral hazard" of insurance: Moral hazard is recognized by most economists (Arrow 1963; Pauly 1968) as the major contributor to market failure in the health care marketplace. *National Commission On The Cost of Medical Care (Budde & Mecher)*

X-ray procedures are exposed to outpatient use (at 80 percent reimbursement), daily room charges in a rational hospital are particularly stuffed with indirect costs.[5] Therefore, the attending physician is pressured, by his failure to appreciate this, into ordering tests rather than waiting to see what time would do for the patient; planning organizations are meanwhile in a deluded frenzy to ration "surplus beds." So long as nothing is done about the underlying indirect costs, however, closing beds or reducing days of stay will merely cause indirect costs to migrate to ancillary services. Charges will escalate even more, if a policy is pursued of writing off the inconvenient 20 percent coinsurance. So, once more, the cost accountant has made innovation possible, but this method of doing so, lacking market restraint, eventually leads to the prohibition of innovation by regulation. (The impression should not be left, however, that scientific innovations like CAT Scanners are the major cause of hospital cost escalation, since it can easily be shown that they are not. The number and size of salaries, and the number and size of buildings would be more realistic areas to examine.)

REMEDY

There is more to say in criticism of the present reimbursement system. But enough. It must be clear that the dual source system is a jerry-built edifice very close to collapsing. A pure retrospective cost reimbursement system would be a still worse disaster, leading first to a few collapses like those of American municipal hospitals, but eventually to lump sum socialism of the Canadian variety, followed in the end by pathetic deterioration of the British sort. Cost reimbursement is a system whereby the tax paying public eventually always demonstrates that it prefers tax reduction to health care, while at the same time refusing to admit it.

We must go back to uniform collection of posted charges. So long as there is pervasive health insurance, it will be difficult to motivate the patient to be concerned about finances when he is

5. There can be even more cycles of reaction and adjustment. Since the daily room-and-board charge is the only visible charge in the mind of the public, and since most people don't pay it anyway, sometimes the room charge is artifically lowered to give a public image of cheapness. The final total bill in such circumstances remains just as large, because other less visible charges are raised.

sick. But the restoration of charges as the basis for all reimbursement should at least motivate the provider to hold down extravagance in order to generate internal profits. It is true that power battles would rage as to whether such internal profits should be applied to scientific innovation, patient amenity, teaching, stockholder dividends, or reduced insurance premiums. But it should not take long for individual hospital distinctiveness to appear,[6] and the sick public can indicate what outcome pleases it best by migrating toward it.

There is an interesting story about how the decision was made to use retrospective cost reimbursement for Medicare and Medicaid. The matter was seriously debated and most of the problems identified. But the overriding consideration quickly emerged that a charge system would immediately flood Medicare with invoices before it could organize a payment system, whereas a retrospective cost-reimbursement system allowed the program a full year to get ready for the audits. Thus the pattern was set. The medical care system would simply have to accomodate itself to the exigencies of administration.

Coinsurance

First, a quick refresher on three terms out of insurance jargon. A *deductible* policy is one in which the insurance carrier only pays a claim of more than a certain amount. The familiar example is the $100 deductible auto accident policy, where the term refers to the fact that the company pays the bill after deducting $100. *Coinsurance* is a type of coverage in which the carrier agrees to pay a percentage of the claim. Here the familiar example is Medicare outpatient (part B) coverage, which pays 80 percent of a claim; the patient is expected to pay 20 percent coinsurance. Both deductible and coinsurance features were designed to create "usage" restraints. The final term is *assignment of benefits,* which is a process by which payment is made directly to the doctor, hospital, or garage mechanic rather than to the person who bought the

6. Assuming planning agencies can be restrained from "regionalizing" away all diversity and competition. Competition and regulation are natural enemies, and regulation is heedless of its enemies.

insurance. The theme here will be that cost reimbursement and assignment have destroyed the utility of deductibles and coinsurance. That is, they have raised medical costs by crippling restraints on "usage."

The reader may not be aware that few hospitals have any incentive to collect the 20 percent coinsurance which is supposedly integral to outpatient Medicare services. The collection costs might be discouragingly high, especially for inexpensive services. Medicare regulations forbid the use of aggressive collection methods, and thereby strongly imply that it is preferable to employ an alternative technique: Write the coinsurance off as uncollectible, and be reimbursed for the resulting bad debt at the year-end cost audit. The linkage of hospital ambulatory services to an inpatient cost reimbursement mechanism thereby confers a considerable competitive advantage over practicing physicians who offer the same services in their offices but who must sustain collection costs and occasional uncollectable losses.

It may also take the reader a moment to follow the logic that outpatient services, officially reimbursed at 80 percent of cost, actually provide a profit over cost. The hospital is reimbursed 80 percent of cost, plus 20 percent of charges (if the coinsurance isn't collected from the patient). Since there is always a markup between costs and charges (varying from 5 to 30 percent), the hospital is then actually receiving 100 percent of cost plus 20 percent of the markup (approximately 106 percent of cost). Since this is one of the three or four areas where a cost-reimbursed hospital can develop a profit, there is a considerable drive to expand outpatient laboratory work. If hospitals thus set about to compete in this area, they seem to the Medicare patient to be "free," while the same service in physicians' offices results in a cash charge to the patient of 20 percent. The physician, in attempting to match the hospital by raising fees and absorbing a 20 percent loss, finds that the "usual, customary, reasonable" limitation system frustrates that response.

Some examples:

The chest X-ray, which Dr. Chamberlain described as costing $5, probably now really costs closer to $18, and so Medicare would reimburse the hospital $14.40 (80 percent of costs), plus $7 (20 percent of the $35 charge) for a total of $21.40. The private X-ray office run by a radiologist in the neighborhood might charge $25, but has to chase the patient for $5 cash and may well result in $20 actually paid. The patient can only see that his $35 hospital X-ray is free, while the "cut-rate" $25 office X-ray costs him $5; indeed, the office radiologist may demand the entire $25, leaving it to the patient to collect $20 from Medicare. The crowning irony of the situation is that the office radiologist may himself believe that he receives $25 in contrast to only $14.40 that the hospital seems to receive. In addition, it is shown in the preceding section of this book that there is shifting of indirect costs away from the radiology department, so that the hospital receives extra money for the chest X-ray disguised as a cost of running the operating room. The effect for society is that private office radiology is rapidly becoming extinct, and the cost to the Medicare program is often higher.

The cardiologist, performing an office electrocardiogram for $25, has a slightly different problem. He, too, must extract $5 cash from the patient (assuming the UCR system[7] allows him a $25 fee, which it may not), while the $45 electrocardiogram at the hospital is "free." Assuming a $10 cost, the hospital receives $17 and adds $28 to the line "free care and reimbursement discounts"[8] in its annual report. As the hospital EKG charge continues to rise, it exerts a powerful psychological effect and causes a general escalation in the price of all electrocardiograms even though the cardiologist may not himself think the high charge is justified. In time, a disproportionate share of his income may come from this source, and his consultation fees fail to keep pace. The result is subsidized distortion of fees in a number of seemingly unrelated areas.

The automated chemistry panel presents a still different problem. But enough. How can we get out of this thicket? One senses that this situation is going to require some coercion to put it to rights, with therefore some risk that the coercion may itself lead to new perversions of incentives. If we could have one wish, what would it be?

It would be *elimination of the use of assignment of benefits on those benefits which have coinsurance features.* There is a temptation to blame cost reimbursement for the present destruction of coinsurance, and there is no doubt it plays an essential role. While

7. UCR means "usual, customary, reasonable." The system provides a flexible ceiling on fees calculated by the flow of charges as received by Medicare.
8. Also known as contractual allowance.

it is also true that some physicians ignore the coinsurance in their own billing, the practice is not nearly so widespread among physicians or commercial laboratories as it is among hospitals; so cost reimbursement is surely some factor.

And there is a temptation to blame gap-filling supplemental insurance such as Blue Cross over-65-Specials. There is obviously something to this reasoning also, since usage restraints are thereby reduced to mere concern about premiums. To make matters worse, the Insurance Commissioner of Pennsylvania has deliberately held down the premiums of the over-65-Special below costs (causing other Blue Cross subscribers to subsidize the elderly). The issue is obviously too politically sensitive to have much prospect of overt correction. The public is at present too much in love with insurance even to examine the matter rationally, so one is led to look elsewhere for workable solutions.

It is here repeated that the easiest administrative method of restoring coinsurance as a usage retraint is to eliminate the assignment option; and this approach seems to be congenial to cultural attitudes about billing and bureaucracy. The patient owns the insurance. He pays a bill and his insurance pays him back. Since he really should not be reimbursed unless he presents a receipted bill, he only gets 80 percent of what he paid. And a side benefit to the program is that the suspicion of fraud is much abated by this routing of money. We will show in Chapter 14, "The Moral Hazard of Third and Fourth Parties," that the general perception among claims departments is that assignment is at least as expensive to administer as indemnity.

Some would say there is one other possible disadvantage to eliminating assignment. The insurance carrier thereby loses the potential to fix fees unilaterally. But that would not seem a great loss to quite everybody. If what we are trying to achieve is to introduce elements of market place discipline, the proposal rests on the proposition that most Americans really do not like to tamper with the market mechanism.

9

Fair Shares

Cindy O'Toole had been a federal civil servant in the Department of Health, Education, and Welfare for ten days, but this was her first day at work. During the other nine days she had been processed through the Civil Service Commission and the personnel department of HEW, her fingerprinting and her physical examination, her placement interviews (with the delays between each step). It had been tedious and confusing; but since each day required only an hour or two of her, it was welcome. In the Washington area it took a lot of time for a newly divorced woman to find a place to live which she could afford. It turned out that she had to take a garden apartment in Virginia that was a forty-minute drive from her new job in Rockville, Maryland. Forty minutes, when she timed it on the Sunday she rented the apartment,became ninety minutes this morning driving with the rush-hour traffic of a one-industry town. There had been no place to park, and she had to pay ten dollars to park in a filling station about a mile from the office building. The building had an enormous parking lot, but the guard would not let her in, even though she could see some empty places very close to the entrance. She was late and it was full. Sorry, lady.

The building was enormous, but until you came near, unobtrusive in the wooded suburban countryside. Fifteen stories high, it didn't look like a skyscraper because its other dimensions were so great. In driving around it, looking vainly for a place to park, she had clocked it as four-tenths of a mile in circumference on the third or fourth circumnavigation. It was really twenty fifteen-story buildings, all glued together. At nearly ten o'clock in the morning, no one was to be seen on the sunny walkways outside. The huge silent pile glowered like a deserted Aztec pyramid in the jungle.

Inside, it was dark. The corridors were narrow, the ceiling low. As Cindy walked down the hall to the elevator (the guard told her that the ground floor was really the fifth floor, so be careful), she could look into some open doorways. Inside were some conventional looking offices with a normal complement of young people looking busy, or typing, or telephoning, or walking around holding a piece of paper. But one important feature closed the whole place in and made it seem unspeakably grim. No windows. You could see from the outside that there were thousands of windows, so somebody had to be near a window. But when you walked through the central corridors you were far, far from daylight, and it looked as though you would probably have to go through five or six rooms before you reached daylight. Ugh. Dante's inferno. Air-conditioned and neon-lighted, but dark and hot.

An intimidating American Indian in a large black forest ranger's hat and string tie held with silver clasp directed her to the office of Mrs. Fremont, who was her new boss. And that was a shock. Mrs. Fremont looked at least a thousand years old, and seemed to weigh only eighty pounds. But she rose from her desk in the inner office and came out to greet her visitor in person. She was wearing extremely thick glasses which grotesquely magnified the appearance of her eyes. Oh God. She has cataracts.

Mrs. Fremont was perfectly charming. It did not take the young woman thirty seconds to realize that here was a person of parts, and there could not possibly be a better person to help a young frightened girl get herself together in a hostile world. "Come in, my dear. I knew you couldn't help but be late on your first day in this anthill, so I went ahead with an appointment with Mr. Behaitcheye, here." For the first time, Ms. O'Toole realized that a little fat man in a lumpy suit had been seated behind the door. "Come in, come in. I understand you worked as an assistant hospital administrator for a year, so maybe you can help us with what we are talking about. Please pour yourself some coffee. Starting tomorrow you can contribute to the coffee fund, but today you are an honored guest.

"I suppose you couldn't get into the parking lot. It's one of the many irritations that have been developed to humiliate your government's loyal employees. You'll find you have to get here an hour early to find a parking space. Another little indignity is signing the time sheet in and out. And the unspeakable stampede in the cafeteria. And the Hatch Act is something you will learn to hate. And the way everybody calls us bureaucrats, so we cluster together even after work. You may well be given power of life and death over large segments of the American public, but Congress sees to it that you don't enjoy it very much."

Mr. Behaitcheye was her old crony, and he applauded her performance. "Sit down, Cindy, and tell us about the real world over there in America. We were just chatting about the reimbursement formula for hospitals."

Ms. O'Toole was greatly encouraged to find a subject she was expert in, so early. "Well, I'm so glad. The present system is terribly unfair."

"Funny you use that word, 'unfair.' All the regulations really require is that we pay hospitals a fair share of their true costs. Unfortunately, nobody knows what is true, and nobody agrees what is fair."

"You're wrong, Jimmy," said Mrs. Fremont. "Nobody agrees what is true and nobody knows what is fair."

"Okay, Tilly, let's put it to our beautiful new acquaintance. How would you define fair reimbursement, Sunshine?"

"I'm not quite sure what you mean."

"All right. Let's say the hospital you worked in has a budget of ten million dollars. Medicare intends to pay its fair share of the ten million but we don't want to pay individual bills. How much do we pay?"

Cindy didn't intend to say anything, and didn't.

"Well, let's say that 40 percent of the patients who are admitted to that hospital have Medicare coverage. So we owe them four million, right?"

"No."

"Why not? That sounds fair to me."

"Medicare patients stay a lot longer than younger patients."

"Very well. You are suggesting that the fair thing is to count up the days of hospitalization. Let us suppose that Medicare subscribers represent 60 percent of the days of care rendered. So we owe them six million dollars, right?"

"Well, that would be better. But I guess it still isn't quite right. Medicare patients are sicker than younger people. They are more demanding. They die."

"Yeah, that's right, some of them are that way. But some others just lie around for weeks recovering from a stroke or a heart attack or a hip operation. How do we know how it is in your old hospital? The chances are, you didn't know yourself when you were there."

"So that's why you pay costs on the basis of charges?"

"That's right, that's why we do. We total up all of the charges which our Medicare patients incur, and the hospital tells us the total of charges that everybody else incurred. We make a ratio, and that's the ratio we pay of your ten million bucks. Charges over charges, applied to costs."

"Well, why don't you just pay the individual charges? Pay each patient's bills, one by one."

"Haw haw! Tilly and I were around in 1965 when this scam was developed. As soon as Lyndon Johnson signed the Medicare Act with sixteen pens, our phone started to ring itself off the wall. Fifty billion old codgers immediately wanted to send us their doctor's bills, and every hospital administrator in the country got on the Metroliner, or whatever we had then, and came down to visit our office; except we didn't have an office. The only thing we could possibly do was whack out a lump sum payment at the end of the year for all of the hospital's Medicare patients by some auditing process; and we didn't even have auditors. It was six months before we could pay anybody a dime, even though every Congressman's secretary called us every morning to ask us why we couldn't do a simple thing like issue a check. If Congress ever passes another one like that, I'm just going to retire to my little boat and catch crabs in the Chesapeake."

"Well, I was only fifteen years old in 1965. You could pay individual charges with computers now."

"You don't know our computers like I know our computers, sweetheart. In fact, you must not know much about any computers."

"I took a course in FORTRAN."

"Oh, God, Tilly. Listen to that. Sunshine, we have four thousand COBOL programmers who would lie down in the street and stop traffic if you used the word FORTRAN. You are much too advanced for us, I'm afraid."

At this, Mrs. Fremont decided enough was enough. "Don't listen to him, Cindy. There aren't many like him around here anymore. Before you came, we were trying to find a way to keep the charges-to-charges, applied-to-costs system from collapsing."

"Why should it collapse?"

"Because the hospital administrators out there in what they call the real world have complete latitude to set the charges at anything they please. So the smart ones raise the prices of items which they notice are used a lot by Medicare patients. If we issue a provider letter on the subject, we may just tip off the dumb ones, and then we are worse off than if we said nothing."

"But you don't pay the individual charges."

"No, we don't. But raising selected charges has the effect of apportioning more of certain costs to Medicare through adjusting the ratio of charges-to-charges, applied to costs. That's what is meant by applied-to-costs."

"So why not develop a fixed fee schedule to prevent funny business in the setting of charges?"

"Tilly!" shouted Mr. Behaitcheye. "She's only been a card-carrying bureaucrat for one day, and she already has the regulatory mentality! Tell them what to do, when to do it, and how much to charge for it. Just swell. Keep it up, Sunshine, and in six months you're going to own this place. They may even give you a window and a place to park."

10

A Message to Big Business

Recently the U.S. Chamber of Commerce studied the question of cost containment in the health field, and urged local chambers to organize data reporting systems for employee health and hospital costs. It is not clear however what employers could do with such information once they had it, since their employees (or unions) are likely to be resentful of intrusion into personal privacy. When the data inevitably demonstrates that some doctors, hospitals, or Health Maintenance Organizations (HMO's) are cheaper than others, the more expensive providers of care would surely assert that you get what you pay for. It would be hard to see how the Chamber of Commerce would prove they were wrong. In any event, the American tradition is for the patient, not his employer, to select his doctor.

A somewhat more productive data analysis for employers would be one which helped them select the cheapest insurance company, or the cheapest health insurance benefit package, for the employee group. While it is true that unions have exerted pressure for enlarged benefit packages, they unite with employers in a desire to get the most benefits for the least health insurance cost. It seems likely that more productive action would result from examination of financial data than medical data, although in both cases it is necessary to be a diligent pupil before the data is intelligible. We here propose that it is worthwhile for unions and employers to understand the ratio of hospital costs to hospital charges. Having understood the matter, the chamber is urged to apply the lesson to local hospitals and individual employee groups.

The examination of internal hospital subsidies is greatly assisted by the existence of an unwieldy document, the SSA-2552. The Medicare agency requires every hospital to complete a 25-page annual financial summary, complete with folded-over pages, and filled with numbers. This document is prepared for a public purpose, and, under the Freedom of Information Act, is available to all who wish to examine it. For the purpose of this chapter, it is possible to ignore all of this document except for column 2 on page 18. On page 18 is found "Worksheet C, The Departmental Cost Distribution." In column 1 will be found the total costs generated by each department during the year (A), together with the total charges generated by that department (B). In column 2, the place where present attention is focused, each department displays the ratio of A divided by B, *the ratio of Cost to Charges*. A quick glance will identify that the ratio is usually less than 1.0, in keeping with the practice of charging more than costs in order to make a "profit." A glance down the line will also likely show a reader that there is a very considerable variation in the ratios from one hospital department to another, and that there are definitely departments with a ratio greater than 1.0, which means that these hospital departments are being subsidized. By you.

The Medicare cost report, available from every hospital, displays the ratio of costs to charges for each revenue-producing department of the hospital. The concept of the ratio is simple enough. In a free enterprise system everyone is accustomed to the idea that the price of things is always a little higher than the cost. The difference is called profit margin, or markup. We are even familiar with the occasional situation where the selling price (charge) is less than the cost; that is called a loss leader.

• Therefore, loss leaders excluded, we would expect the normal ratio of costs to charges to be approximately .90, allowing about a 10 percent profit for bad debts, charity, etc.

• Furthermore, we would expect the individual departments of the hospital to display a cost-to-charge ratio which is relatively uniform, and fairly close to the overall total for the hospital.

• Notice that the important issue is not how close the ratio is to unity (1.0) but rather how uniform the ratios are between departments.

• A great many people assume that, if the cost-charge ratio is less than 1.0 and a profit is therefore generated, any insurance company which pays charges must have higher premiums than an insurance company which pays "costs." Such an inference is not justified in theory, and is quite clearly incorrect in certain circumstances. The premium reflects all of the expenses of the insurance company, not just the hospital payments. Subsidy of nongroup individual subscribers by group subscribers is a major example of the equalizers affecting health insurance premiums.

• The following figures for cost-to-charge ratios were taken from an actual hospital's Medicare cost report. The report, but not necessarily the numbers, is typical of most hospitals, although there is a great deal of individual variation between hospitals. The important things to notice are the nonuniformity of departments, and the separability of hospital departments into two distinct classes:

RATIO OF COSTS TO HOSPITAL CHARGES BY DEPARTMENT

SUBSIDIZED BY BLUE CROSS, MEDICARE, MEDICAID	(RATIO)	SUBSIDIZED BY COMMERCIAL INSURANCE AND CASH PATIENTS	(RATIO)
Operating Room	1.02	X-Ray	.74
Short Procedure	1.20	Isotopes	.68
Labor & Delivery	1.32	Laboratory	.69
Anaesthesia	1.19	Oxygen	.59
Physical Therapy	1.38	EKG	.22
Daily Room Charge	1.22	EEG	.54
Intensive Care Unit	1.25	Medical Supplies	.46
(This classification is the author's.)		Drugs	.58

Finally, one dare not assume that the cost-to-charge ratio for a department is reflected in every service performed by that department. The ratio comes about by the cost accountant assigning indirect costs to those departments which have the best cost reimbursement experience. At the same time, charges are raised on those items most likely to be paid for in cash, within the perceived limits of ability to pay. Charges tend to be closely examined on common items like blood counts and chest X-rays, while uncommon tests and services tend to be too much trouble to examine frequently in close detail. Therefore, there are often bargains in rarely used services whose charges have not been raised in some time. Finally, there are items which can be charged off as bad debts if unpaid by a Medicare patient. Under this heading are personal items like television sets, or uncollected 20 percent coinsurance on ambulatory services; for setting charges on these items, there are no rules.

How to Play the Game

The free-market, or Adam Smith, theory is presumably highly regarded by the Chamber of Commerce. The theory supposes that every rational person will press his own interest and advantage to the point where he comes into equilibrium with the rest of the community, who are simultaneously acting on their behalf. It must be clear that the hospital financial and reimbursement system strongly endorses the "every man for himself" philosophy. What follows are a few suggestions for the business world to play the hospital game with a little more success than has been demonstrated in the past. Perhaps if it does, the community at large will benefit as a new equilibrium is set.

• Notice that a cost/charge ratio greater than unity (1.0) means a loss leader. If your insurance company pays charges, it is paying less than another company which is paying costs. If you have insurance which pays costs, the reverse is true.

• Notice that the benefit package of an insurance company should heavily include the use of those hospital departments which are loss-leaders according to the type of insurance you have. Select benefits in the left column if you use a commercial carrier. Select benefits in the right column if you have Blue Cross, or change carriers if you want the benefit.

• Notice that the cost-reimbursing insurance companies create motivations to include a large number of ambulatory benefits, since they get a bargain on such services. However, if they were restrained from this, they might be forced to resist the cost escalation of inpatient-intensive services, which means they would resist the current escalation of indirect costs. Since the root cause of hospital inflation is the rampant growth of indirect costs, it is possible that restricting Blue Cross to in-patient reimbursement would slow the spiral.

• If an employer intends to be serious about playing the hospital game, he needs to know what kind of services his own employees are using. He also needs to know what the particular cost / charge quirks are at the local hospitals where most of his employees find themselves from time to time. It is easy to imagine one employer with 80 percent of his employees women under the age of thirty, while another employer mostly might have nothing but middle-aged male employees. A new business will have young active employees, and older businesses may have pensioners to consider. Climate makes a difference, and occupational hazards must be considered. So, what's good for one employer isn't necessarily good for others, or necessarily good after the business has grown for ten years. And the hospital cost accountant, by the way, isn't going to be asleep as things change over time.

• It would require a rather sophisticated data system for an employer group (or even an insurance company) to analyze its experience in terms of hospital departmental usage. So a simpler conceptual approach is suggested. The departments with a high cost / charge ratio tend to be used by surgeons and surgical special-ties. Conversely, the nonsurgical physicians (internists, pediatri-cians, psychiatrists, family practitioners) tend to use most heavily the hospital departments which have a low cost / charge ratio. There is no conspiracy at work; it just happens to work out that way as a result of independent stresses which have been discussed earlier in this section.

So, it would appear that the patients of nonsurgeons subsidize patients who have surgery. Somewhat true, although the situation is more complicated.

Both Blue Cross and the commercial carriers employ an analytic system for large employee groups, known as experience rating. For reasons of practicality, Blue Cross conducts group experience rating on the basis of charges incurred (even though the plan pays costs, not charges). The commercial carriers experience-rate on the basis of charges, too, but they actually pay the charges. So, an experience-rated group gains nothing by switching carriers so long as the experience rating continues to be based on hospital charges.

The premium they pay will reflect a subsidy of surgical patients by nonsurgical ones.

But there is another class of patients for whom the reverse is true. The nongroup individual subscribers to Blue Cross likewise have a diversion of premium money toward surgery, while at the same time receiving a subsidy from the group subscribers. It is difficult to tell whether the combined effect is positive or negative for the surgical patients. But the nonsurgical, nongroup subscribers are certainly getting a bargain. Until someone figures out a way to force subscribers to belong to a group, a company should think twice about forming one. Decreased benefit package? Buy an excess major medical policy and forget it.

• Of all the subsidies which characterize this giant medical financial equilibrium, the greatest is on the basis of the age of the subscriber. It scarcely needs proof to recognize that young subscribers do not have the same health costs as older ones, but they often pay the same premium. All health insurance plans would do well to devise a system of vesting before competition exploits this inherent weakness and topples the structure. A movement by entire groups into nongroup would eventually reach an equilibrium, but a selective movement of young subscribers to step-rated[1] competitors or self-insurance would start a spiral which could be very drastic, indeed.

• Finally, there is one other recourse which subscribers could take to the situation wherein nonsurgical hospital patients subsidize surgical ones, while experience-rating prevents them from doing much about it. The recourse would be to seek care outside of a hospital. For example, nowadays, there is not much difference between a first-class nursing home and a hospital, except that you can't do much surgery in the nursing home.

---

1. The premium goes up in steps, usually in five- or ten-year age brackets.

11

Pit Stop: An Interim Summary

In an earlier chapter, we asked the question: Why do hospitals cost so much? By looking at the issues from a macroeconomic and then from a medical descriptive point of view, we derived two answers:

1. They cost so much because of the moral hazard of health insurance, intentionally encouraged by society to disseminate universal access to modern health care.

2. They cost so much because of a list of good and bad things (mostly good) which were medicine's response to the public mandate that money was to be no object.

After reviewing the cost accounting and reimbursement situation, two more answers can be added:

3. They cost so much because the situation has permitted an extensive network of subsidies. It cannot be said whether these subsidies are good or bad until they come out into the open and receive public approval or disapproval. By and large, no one elected the people who have created these subsidies, but they are decent people and they may well be correct in their view of what the public wants.

4. They cost so much because there are so many indirect costs. If you want to know where the bodies are buried, take a look at the indirect costs, which are 50 percent of the costs of even a small rural hospital. They are often 70 percent of the costs of a metropolitan teaching hospital.

We now turn our attention to the last major component of the hospital cost problem, the financing and proliferation of capital facilities. That is, hospital buildings.

12

Building Mrs. O'Leary's Hospital

To understand hospital finances, one must understand the pivotal role of the hospital building. A hospital might be growing in financial strength or it might be using up its heritage, but one would have trouble telling which was the case without examination of its real estate situation. Everything about hospital building value is debatable, since the specialized structure is not worth much for other purposes. But there are formulas used by the banking and real estate fraternities to estimate values, and certain reimbursement rules create tangible value. We begin with a consideration of residual value.

RESIDUAL VALUES

The best example of residual value would be the Pine Street buildings of America's first hospital. The original building of the Pennsylvania Hospital maintained an average census of 150 patients from 1755 to 1965. In all probability, the building was completely paid for during the eighteenth century, and it can be estimated that during the following years it housed ten or eleven million days of patients care without any capital cost or debt service. True, there were several renovations, and an old structure requires more expensive maintenance than a new building. But most hospital structures do have a useful life considerably in excess of the arbitrary reimbursement definition of useful life, which is forty years. Such residual useful life is a "profit" which the institution realizes after forty years. It is also an asset which is sacrificed whenever the structure is demolished to make way for a replacement.

DEPRECIATION: FUNDED, UNFUNDED,
INVESTED, OR SPENT

Nevertheless, in practical affairs there must be decisions, and so a new hospital building is assumed to have a useful life of forty years. The construction costs are spread over that period of time, so each generation of patients will pay its share. At the same time, prudent management recognizes that the building will eventually have to be replaced. Each patient should be charged his share of one year's "depreciation," which is assumed each year to be a fortieth of the construction cost. The money will not be needed for many years for new building purposes, and during that time many other worthy purposes will appear. The hospital has a choice of the path of fiscal virtue ("funded" depreciation), or the path of waywardness ("unfunded" depreciation). They can save it, or they can spend it.

While hospitals may voluntarily fund depreciation, even full funding of the original construction cost will not guarantee self-sufficiency. During periods of inflation, the original construction price of a building cannot reasonably be expected to replace the structure forty years later; indeed, it may then amount to less than 20 percent of the replacement cost. Therefore, depreciation sinking funds must not just be stored; they must be successfully invested. The temptation to dissipate even the investment proceeds must be resisted, except for short intervals, since only untaxed compound interest can keep up with inflation of construction costs.

(For the past six years, Federal Reserve policy has maintained interest rates below the rate of inflation. That is definitely not the traditional relationship between the two, and the safety of our economy depends on a return to a rate of interest greater than the annual loss due to inflation.)

As a side issue, proprietary hospital chains can convert their depreciation to a contemporary basis by selling hospitals to each other, and using the sale price as the basis of depreciation rather than the construction cost. Although their nonprofit competitors criticize them, this probably is a fair practice, which balances to some degree the taxability of their investment dividends.

Depreciaton is a confusing subject to talk about, because even if you understand what it is, you may get lost when hospital insiders use the term carelessly. When a building depreciates, it slowly loses value; it wears out. This is the physical process of depreciation. In addition, there is a conceptual depreciation in which the usefulness of the building is gradually being lost, even though the physical structure looks pretty good and has an appreciable salvage value. It is the conceptual loss of useful life which is the kind of depreciation that accountants try to estimate by their formulas. It quite obviously is a matter of opinion, no matter how honest the accountants try to be.

A prudent institution might try to set aside a replacement sum each year according to a schedule which would accumulate enough money to replace the building when the time comes to do so. However, in an inflationary era, it is almost impossible to do this with accuracy, and the process of saving up to be able to buy later has been largely abandoned. Rather, it has become more attractive to borrow the money to build a new building, build it, and then pay off the loan over the useful life of the building. Buy now, pay later.

Therefore, depreciation nowadays is spoken of both as a cost and as a revenue source. It is a cost, because some bank or bond fund must be paid; the term amortization is equivalent. Depreciation is also revenue, because the reimbursement agencies recognize that their patients are helping to wear out the building, and they pay their share. The charges to those few patients who pay charges should include an amount calculated to pay their fair share of the depreciation cost. To repeat: Depreciation is both a cost, and also a source of revenue.

However, the dollar amounts of depreciation cost and depreciation revenue are not the same in any given year, even though the totals are indeed equal over the life of the building. In early years, depreciation revenue is greater than depreciation cost, and in later years the cost is greater than the revenue. This is a very important concept, and it is unfamiliar to many nonhospital financial people who deal with mortgages every day.

The quirk in the hospital mortgage field lies in the fact that interest costs and repayment of principal ("depreciation") are reimbursed at two different speeds by third parties like Medicare. Interest is fully reimbursed in the year it is incurred. Naturally, interest costs get less every year of the mortgage, going from a large amount the first year to a very small amount in the last year of the mortgage. (But, who cares, because they are transparent, being immediately and fully reimbursed the same year.)

So interest costs get less each year, and the repayment of principal stays the same? No, that's wrong. Interest costs get less, all right, but the repayment of principal to the bank gets larger each year. The bank arranges the necessary arithmetic so that the total monthly mortgage payment which it receives is exactly the same throughout the life of the mortgage. Surely this is a familiar subject to our mortgaged society. You make the same payment every month, but in the first month it is almost all interest, while in the very last month it is almost all principal.

Although the depreciation cost (repayment of loan principal) starts low and goes high, the depreciation revenue is a steady medium amount the whole time. The revenue is based on a "forty-year straight line depreciaton" which means 2½ percent of the principal every year for forty years. To oversimplify, you generate a cash surplus in the first half of the mortgage, and you are in a cash shortage the last half. If you saved (funded) the surplus from the early years of the loan, you just pay it out in the late life of the loan (and you can keep the interest which the early-life surplus earned, as a little bonus). Yes, it's true. You get paid back a little more than it cost you to build the building. If you don't have any bad debt losses you make a profit, just building away. But you almost certainly do have some bad debts, so it isn't unfair to garner the interest.

What is bad, unspeakably bad, is to spend the early-life cash surplus on cakes and ale (unfunded depreciation), because how are you going to pay back the cash crunch in the late life of the loan? Mephistopheles in a three-piece suit whispers a suggestion: You could just build a second building and apply its early-life cash surplus to the late-life cash deficit of the first building. And you could later build a third building, or a fourth. But like any other chain letter, you know it will collapse. You don't know when or how, but it will eventually collapse.

The foregoing is, as most readers would suspect, an oversimplification. Most mortgages only run for twenty years, so every hospital has a cash shortage from construction, about seven to fifteen years out. They will have a twenty-year cash surplus during years twenty to forty (when the Medicare reimbursement runs out). After year forty, there is the salvage value of the building, or its residual utility value, if you want to keep on using it. The land the building rests on doesn't count. Land doesn't wear out.

There are further quirks growing out of the special features of tax-exempt municipal bond funding and refunding. For example, it wouldn't hurt a bit to insist on competitive bidding for the under-writing and legal costs. It wouldn't hurt any to have the SEC pass approval on the prospectus.[1] Finally, it gives a very small investor great pleasure to give some advice to the very large institutional investors in municipal bonds: Before you invest, investigate.

THE ROLE OF DONATED MONEY

Charitable donations are not nearly as important for hospital building programs as they once were, but if available they permit a more imaginative financial structure. Under the old system, a potential large donor would have it explained that his donation could really be spent twice. It would build the building, and then the depreciation reimbursement would appear later as revenue, to be spent a second time. It might be spent the second time on cakes and ale, or it might be used to build a second building in the future. And a third building, and a fourth, when each capital expenditure is eventually returned intact as depreciation reim-bursement. It is true that inflation of building costs creates an attrition of the building fund, but that is offset somewhat by the accumulation of residual and salvage values.

At the present time, revolving capital building funds are more likely to be created by aggregating nonpatient revenues and small donations without much consultation with the donors. Probably the most important objection to this system is the way desirable current programs are sacrificed on the altar of facility expansion. There is nothing quite so hard and uncharitable as a hospital trying to accumulate a building fund. To the extent that the original donors might have thought they were supporting charity, their presumed attitudes should be respected.

Depreciation is a "cost." That is, the reimbursement agencies allow the depreciation allotment to be listed among the legitimate

---

1. On the other hand, the bonding authority may well insist on a sinking fund.

costs of the institutions, and reimbursed during the year incurred, in the proportion that the clients of the particular third party used the institution during the year. Naturally, charity patients are unable to provide their share of depreciation, and force the institution to consider less than full funding. That is, the hospital "dips into depreciation." Because truly poor patients since 1966 have been covered by Medical Assistance, and since 94 percent of Americans now have some health coverage, an appreciable proportion of bad debts come from patients who have run out of benefits. Therefore, the issue causes considerable resentment against the reimbursement agency which covered the patient up to the benefit cutoff.

FIFTEEN YEARS, THE DANGEROUS AGE

Any banker who places a mortgage on a hospital takes risks which he would never take on an ordinary business loan, and counts on the indispensibility of the institution making up for its unsalability as collateral. He can hardly be blamed for limiting the term of the mortgage to twenty years, comfortably short of the fortieth year when the reimbursement agencies stop making depreciation payments. But the banker's prudence causes a foreseeable cash shortage for the hospital, since a repayment of one twentieth is going to be more expensive than one fortieth can support. The peculiar combination of mortgage and reimbursement causes a predictable cash shortage for the hospital during the fifteenth to twentieth years. The long and short of it is that a new building gives a hospital a cash *surplus* during the first few years, a cash *shortage* after 15 years, a *surplus* again from 20 to 40 years, and a *residual profit* after 40 years.

Since these curves can be reasonably predicted, it makes sense to build or replace the hospital in sections, with the cash surplus of a new building offsetting the cash deficit of a 15-year-old building. Unfortunately, the new building may require the demolition of a still older structure which is in the cash surplus (20 to 40 years) or "pure gravy" (40-plus) stages. A balance must then be struck between the loss of this asset and the advantages of the new building, such as its ability to attract patients in a competitive environment, reduced maintenance costs, creation of an eventually more valuable paid-up property, better service to the community and greater employee satisfaction. Most Americans would hold that a new building is generally superior to an old one; OSHA (Occupational Safety and Health Administration) and the Joint Commission for the Accreditation of Hospitals certainly believe so. In addition to prosaic reasons, there are obviously hospitals which need to be built in response to desperate local shortages of beds and facility. Still, it cannot be denied that one of the important elements of increasing cost of hospital care has been the rather marked shortening of useful life of capital structures.

There are observers who raise some even more disturbing points about hospital construction finance. There is concern that the cash shortages of the amortization schedule will themselves be sufficiently threatening that some institutions, who have spent away their early depreciation, might be driven to consider a new building purely as a source of cash to pay earlier debts. This would of course be a hopeless venture. Quite aside from the unneeded construction which would result, the financial quicksand would be such that only the government could conceivably rescue the situation. Those who fear government ownership of hospitals must be concerned that such predicaments must be prevented; a fundamental revision of the system of reimbursement is not too great a price to pay.

THE ROLE OF DONATED MONEY

Meanwhile, we have the system of "cost" reimbursement, and we have municipal bond finances. Each has a bearing, in different ways, on contributed donations to building fund drives. Donations represent a much smaller proportion of the cost of a hospital building than they formerly did; but the seed-money role of contributions is still critical. Bankers want the term of the mortgage to be less than the useful life of the building; they also want a down payment. If the hospital can generate enough cash for a down payment, the building is as good as paid for. A donor, in turn, finds that his contribution serves doubly when given to a building drive: paying for the building, and generating depreciation revenue to be spent a second time. A distinction can thus be made between borrowed funds, which must be repaid, and donated or "found" money, which need not be repaid. If the hospital spends the depreciation on borrowed money, it is on a one-way trip to disaster; donated money was meant to be spent, and spent twice over. Doubly spent money can be generated by means other than donation. In many hospitals, nonpatient income (parking fees, rental on doctors offices, investment dividends, etc.) can amount to 10 percent of the operating budget of the hospital. It could be argued that the most productive use of such money is to provide a down payment on a new building, being later recycled into still more building as the depreciation is "earned."

MUNICIPAL BOND FINANCING

A more "modern" system of construction finance is to induce the local municipality to issue bonds on behalf of the hospital expansion, since municipalities have the right to pay interest which exempts the purchaser from federal income taxes. Such interest rates are generally one or two percent lower than ordinary taxable-bond interest rates, and can be fairly viewed as receiving a federal subsidy. They can also be issued for the full construction price if the underwriter will permit it, thus freeing the hospital of the need to generate a down payment. This last feature comes about from the fact that a bond is related to the ability of the institution to generate future income, rather than being based on the underlying value of the chattel asset as is the case with a mortgage. Other features:

1. Donations by physician staff members are mostly valuable as a sign to the investment community that the medical staff will supply patients to generate reimbursement to service the bond.

2. Ownership of the bonds is scattered among investors across the country, who know much less about what they are supporting than the local bank would know about its mortgagee. Indeed, the bank is very likely to have an officer who is a trustee of the hospital. Obviously, such intermingled interests can have both good and bad effects.

3. Small investors often assume that the prospectus and underwriting of municipal bonds are overseen and guarded by the SEC. Unfortunately, such is not the case. Whether or not the underwriting and legal fees are open to competitive bidding is a

matter for local discretion. As in the case of bankers, the participation of legal and underwriting firms with connections to the trustees can have effects which are both good and bad, depending on whether the financing is seen as a risky charity or a riskless plum.

4. Quite often the period for redemption of the bond is longer than the normal term of a mortgage. The "squeeze" on cash flow at fifteen years is thus relieved, along with the need for down payment capital. Cash excess at the beginning of the building life is enhanced because a greater proportion of the debt service is interest, and interest is reimbursable immediately.

5. It should be noticed that the instant reimbursability of interest means that hospitals are peculiarly indifferent to interest rates. They would be wise to exercise voluntary restraint of construction at times when the Federal Reserve is attempting to cool inflation by raising interest rates; otherwise, public resentment may precipitate regulatory restraint. If this danger is avoided, however, there are cost advantages to building at times when the construction industry is underemployed. Furthermore, if interest rates should subsequently fall below the bond coupon, the bonds can be called and reissued at the lower rate. While the effect of refinancing is to increase the total principal which must eventually be repaid, it may be more important to extend the time before the fifteen-year cash shortage appears, since refinancing resets the clock.

6. There are, of course, problems. The defaults of the city of Cleveland have warned investors that municipal bonds may not be totally safe. The wrenching decline in bond prices following the revelation of New York City's problems was an earlier object lesson. The eternal earning power of hospitals is predicated on eternal cost reimbursement; some may feel the premise is questionable. The demographics and health characteristics of a city forty years in the future will probably be unpredictably different, as 1978 was different from 1938. And finally, the necessary involvement with local municipal politicians may be too close, for everyone's taste, at the time when necessary cooperation and permission is being sought in floating the bond issue.

SUMMARY

The present financing climate has quite obviously assisted a major boom in hospital construction. No one can deny that one of the results has been an increase in the cost of hospital care. It is quite difficult to know whether there is serious hidden financial weakness as a result of overreaching. If so, a step toward government takeover has been made. If not, the following changes can be seen as the hidden "profit":

1. Air conditioning has become standard.
2. There are fewer occupants in a room, leading to greater privacy, but increasing nursing costs.
3. The Life Safety Code (OSHA) has been enforced.
4. There has been a major increase in the ratio of bathrooms to patients.
5. The average useful life of the building has been drastically shortened. Administrative staffs have had to be increased to cope with the turnover.
6. The hospitals possess a much larger financial asset on which to coast if periods of fiscal stringency should face them with long bleak periods such as the one British medicine has had for the past thirty years. The great danger is that, in guarding against the worst, hospitals may precipitate the worst, by discrediting themselves through overexpansion which eventually anyone can see, or bankruptcies whose cause will eventually be widely understood. Tax-exempt public service monopolies, the majority of whose income comes from tax-supported public programs, and whose capital financing is based on tax-exempt municipal bonds (if you accept that definition of hospitals)—are not in a good position to resist a public takeover when they get into financing trouble.

To allow that to happen is to create socialized medicine without taking the traditional intermediate step of nationalized health insurance.

13

Going to the Wall

Seventh floor: Eleven o'clock in the morning. Fine old investment banking firm, Wall Street. The receptionist sits in the center of a large doughnut of a desk in front of the bank of elevators, near the intersection of two corridors, both thickly carpeted. To her left is a large enclosure of darkened glass which creates one side of a conference room. There are drapes which can be pulled across the inside of the dark glass, but they are open. The two men seated at the conference table seem to glow like figures on a screen surrounded by darkness, Rembrandt portraits. Chiarascuro.

A plump red-faced junior partner of the firm, Mr. Dow, is talking with an associate of the firm, Mr. Harlow O'Toole. Dow is forty-two. O'Toole, thirty-four, is engaged chiefly in the flotation of municipal bonds, a major activity of the firm in recent months. They are mostly killing time until their guests arrive and they have been talking business for half an hour.

"Should we take them to the partner's dining room for lunch?" asks O'Toole.

"Oh, hell, I don't know," replies Mr. Dow, "the food is so damned rich and I'm trying to lose a few pounds. I'd really rather eat over at the Tavern, where you can relax a little. But it's true that out-of-towners are always eager to tell the folks that they ate in a top-floor private dining room on Wall Street. They can say that somebody like Bernie Baruch was at the next table."

Mr. O'Toole understood what he was really hearing. No liquor was allowed in the executive dining room, and there were men waiters. However, he hadn't been elected to a junior partnership yet, and he knew better than to get fresh. "Well maybe they have other plans for lunch. We can play it by ear. But if they really want to eat here, why don't we do it? After all, you know, never kick a man when he's up."

Mr. Dow nodded. "But you please remember, eating in that dining room is like having a belly button. Everybody has one, but nobody wants two."

"Say, boss," said O'Toole to open a discussion, "I hope you noticed how the hospital bonding issues are leading the pack in the tax-exempts this month. Pretty good for a new concept, right?"

"So what else is there?" answered Dow. "Since the interstate highway system, nobody's building turnpikes, the end of the baby boom ended bonds for school buildings, mass transit is a fizzle, and New York City plus Proposition Thirteen chopped the General Obligations. What does that leave? Airports and hospitals, and not many airports."

"Well, okay, but if all you have is a hammer, you might just as well treat everything like a nail. If it's the only game in town, let's be players."

For a moment, Dow didn't answer. "Some of those things bother me. You remember that teaching hospital we floated in March? My God, after you and I went through their books, I had to give myself soda bicarb."

"Yes, and what happened?" replied O'Toole. "You know we brought the news back to the senior partners and old Joe Jones told us to take a chance on thirty million. 'Very prestigious hospital,' he says. So we put everything in the prospectus, warts and all, and brought it out by 9 A.M. By noon we had ninety million in purchase orders."

"So no one read a two-hundred-page prospectus," answered Dow.

"So what else is new? If that's the way banks and insurance companies like to buy bonds, I suppose we can't kick, but it worries me. Any day now, one of those hospitals is going to go down the tube, and then the investment community is going to say, 'Well, we always knew you have to be able to tell a good one from a bad one.' And then the next thing they will ask is, 'By the way, how are we supposed to tell a good one from a bad one?' "

"By that time, you will be retired, and the younger generation can take over," said O'Toole, venturing a little. "You know how these things generate a surplus the first five to ten years."

Dow looked out the window toward the church steeple at the end of the street. "If you ask me, it's like playing leapfrog with a unicorn. . . . Two guys just got off the elevator, are they our guests?"

Mr. Wynne and Mr. Morris waited in front of the conference room glass wall while the receptionist announced them, and Mr. O'Toole, who had met them before, hurried out to greet them and escort them into the large, luminous room.

"Welcome, welcome, gentlemen. I suppose you have already found out that New York isn't a Mecca, it just smells like one! We just had a fresh cup of coffee while we conferred for an hour about your new issue and other matters. Won't you have some coffee? This is Mr. Dow, the partner assigned to your issue."

Mr. Dow was careful to take charge of the meeting from the first moment. "Please be comfortable, gentlemen. Mr. O'Toole always talks like that. He's the sort of guy who always leaves a breeze after he passes."

It emerged that Mr. Morris and Mr. Wynne had developed a concern about the proposed bond issue for their hospital, and as trustees had decided to go directly to the investment bankers themselves to talk it over.

Mr. Dow gave them a wan smile. "There are always risks in anything, I guess. But if you should get into trouble with these revenue bonds, you sure would have an awful lot of company. The investment community has taken very warmly to these issues, and after all you are providing an absolutely vital commodity. It's hard for me to imagine the country permitting the hospitals to close."

Mr. Wynne nodded. "My father used to say that if you owe a bank five thousand dollars and can't repay it, you have a problem. But if you owe the bank five million dollars and can't repay it, the bank is the one with the problem."

Mr. Morris wasn't so sure. "Now look. Bonds are based on revenues projected forty years into the future. They can't possibly be as conservative a lien as a twenty-year mortage."

"Oh, I don't agree," interjected O'Toole. "You are absolutely assured of 100 percent depreciation, no matter what payment mechanism our faithful public servants devise in the future. Building costs can go nowhere else but up in the future, so the investment looks better and better every year you look back on it. If you want my opinion, you could build a Hyatt Regency for the Salvation Army and depreciate it out just fine."

Mr. Morris persisted. "It makes me uncomfortable to get into unfunded depreciation. It's like New York City and its problems. It lets you live beyond your means for a while, but later . . ."

Mr. Dow was gently reassuring. "I know exactly what you are saying, and I have my worries about some bonds that our less scrupulous competitors have brought out. If I were you, I would insist on fully funding the depreciation. That would be a very prudent position for a trustee. And your perceptiveness would be a good example for other hospitals, believe me."

Mr. O'Toole followed up. "And if you need the flexibility for cash flow, it's always there because you funded the depreciation voluntarily. It's not as if the government stuck its big nose into your affairs. I suppose you heard that gag about the way to make absolutely sure that crime won't pay is to have the government take it over."

Mr. Morris said nothing, and looked down at his shoes. Mr. Dow noticed the reluctance and began to purr. "A hospital is like any other business; it has to be efficient to survive. We looked over your books and your conservatism really pleased me. You should have seen one hospital we looked over this spring. They had so many employees they could have applied for statehood. But that must be exceptional, thank God. The great market restraint on hospitals is that most of their products are pretty uncomfortable."

Mr. Wynne smiled. "Well, there's always going to be criticism. Fred Allen used to say that if criticism had power to harm you, the skunk would be extinct."

Mr. Morris was starting to loosen up, but something remained on his mind. "Do you imagine that every hospital in the country could float these bonds? It just doesn't seem possible that everyone could do it."

"You are absolutely right, sir," said O'Toole. "In this country we are anxious for the greatest good for the greatest number. But believe me, the truly greatest number is always Number One."

Mr. Morris smiled. "Yes, Benjamin Franklin used to say that one today is worth two tomorrows."

At that, Mr. Dow stood up. "Would you gentlemen care to join us for lunch in the partners' dining room? It's just upstairs, and the food is really pretty good."

14

The Moral Hazard of Third and Fourth Parties

The two main parties involved in health care are the patient and the provider of care. They have their business to do, and neither party likes to be worried about anything but health care at the time of the encounter. Health insurance helps both of them do what is to be done without concern about finances, at least at the time of the illness. Unfortunately, the use of insurance brings two more parties into a four-cornered transaction. The third party is an insurance company or government agency, and the fourth party is often an employer or government who pays the premiums. The price the medical system pays for relief from financial concern at the time of illness is both financial and substantive. There is intrusion of pressure from the third and fourth parties to accomodate their own particular needs. Insurance administration is also not free; the administrative overhead cost for all third-party reimbursement for health care was over $10 billion in 1978.

The substantive price to be paid is yielding to the convenience or weakness of the third parties, who in turn are very responsive to the pressures of the employer or government. Who pays the piper calls the tune, and neither the third party nor the fourth party is exclusively concerned about health care.

If the third party is a for-profit corporation, it will have some concern about administrative overhead. But even a for-profit insurance company has reason to tolerate high billings in order to maintain the essential role of insurance. The $10 billion has some moral hazard components, too.

In this chapter, we discuss the unfortunate consequences of

overextending the range of benefits of insurance coverage, the short-cut of paying the provider of care directly instead of involving the patient, and a fourth-party attempt to eliminate the third party.

The Benefit Package and Fourth Party Payers

An insurance policy is a contract in which a client obligates himself to pay a premium. In return, the insurance company defines a list of circumstances in which it will pay up. That list of circumstances, called a benefit package, would normally be limited to those risks which were serious enough to warrant the sales and administrative costs of the insurance mechanism, and a prudent buyer would start insuring the worst risks first.

Unfortunately, a heavy proportion of health insurance is paid for by employers or government (the fourth parties), and that fact immediately reverses the incentive of the insured client. With someone else paying the premium, it is desirable to have coverage provisions be as generous as possible. During the past thirty years, there has been a steady broadening of prevailing health insurance benefit coverages.

When government is the paying fourth party, a total incentive-reversal occurs. When employers are paying on behalf of employees, however, both sides recognize that the employer regards fringe benefits as a labor cost. If he pays more in fringes, he will pay less in wages. In the case of employer-paid health insurance, the stimulus to broaden coverage provisions (i.e., raising premium levels) is not the fact that the employer pays the bill; the stimulus is the fact that the employee is not required to pay income tax on nonwage compensation of this sort. As inflation has promoted everyone into higher progressive income tax brackets, the compensation may be worth 30 to 50 percent more to the employee when it is received as an enlargement of health insurance coverage. If it is worth more to the employee, it seems correspondingly more attractive to the employer to pay him in that manner. So, both employers and employees share a financial incentive to broaden the coverage provisions as much as possible. While there is no question this is a blatant tax loophole, the likelihood of elected politicians opposing something supported by both management and labor is very small indeed.

Whenever elected governments paint themselves into such corners politically, there is a standard way out. A blue ribbon commission gets appointed to make a study and write a "white paper" which describes the cost of the tax loophole, and proposes several means by which it could be closed, or some way in which the courts could be encouraged to "legislate" a solution. Presumably, some other blue ribbon commission would have to examine the cost of overextending the benefits into claims so small that the claims processing would be as complicated as the medical process it pays for. It might take several white papers before public awareness reached the point where something could be done, and whatever could be done would probably only be a step toward closing the loophole. The last chapter of this book proposes a way of addressing overextended health benefits without confronting the tax loophole. It is possible that I exaggerate the obstacles to achieving unpopular but necessary tax legislation, but I doubt it.

Now let's look for a moment at the position of organized labor on first-dollar coverage of comprehensive health benefits.

Organized labor has never liked deductibles and coinsurance, and part of this feeling is a genuine concern that the health of union members might suffer if medical usage restraints were imposed. Walter Reuther is said to have felt very deeply that the UAW (United Auto Workers) had a social responsibility to its members and dependents to protect them against their own occasional foolishness. No one had to give Reuther a lesson on the sad irresponsibility of some people in squandering earnings which the UAW had fought to get for them. Now that the Auto Workers have a 1980 contract paying close to $11 an hour, many union officers feel it is in the best interest of many union members to have enforced saving against a rainy day. The longshoremen, who in 1979 received $6.10 an hour in fringe benefits on top of their $10 wage, feel the same way. Although union officers are usually very conservative people, the rhetoric of class struggle is never far below the surface when fringe benefits are discussed. Their employers are not going to argue with them, and their congressmen won't either. Out of fairness, congress might well extend the tax loophole to everyone who does not now enjoy it, but it is hard to see the loophole being eliminated unless something very substantial is offered in its place (see the last chapter).

Meanwhile, the health insurance benefit package gets extended every year, and every extension is more dubious than the last. Extending the coverage of Medicaid to out-patient drugs is a very popular proposal among the elderly, and one can easily see why it might be so. Surprisingly, those druggists who have had experience with free drug programs under Medicaid are quite reluctant to see more free programs created even though they see well enough that it would increase their business. Some of them tell me that 70 percent of their business now consists of dispensing tranquilizers to people on free programs; birth control pills are a poor second. Home nursing care also sounds like an attractive alternative to hospital or nursing home care until you learn of charges of $45 per visit; once again, it is surprising how many visiting nurses are critical of making their services a seemingly free benefit. Psychiatrists are similarly torn because, knowing how limited they sometimes are by a very sick patient's resources, they also are aware of the flood of hypochondriasis awaiting the opening of the insurance door.

The argument is frequently heard that patients might be forced into hospitals for treatment which would be covered with insurance only there. That sounds plausible, but it is surprising how infrequently it actually occurs. For the most part, effective out-patient alternatives do not exist in urban ghettos, and the social situation is such that hospitalization is often required for reasons that have nothing to do with reimbursement for services. Hospitals were originally founded in this country because of a recognition of the facts of indigent home situations. Until this century, middle-class people expected to be treated at home—and they seldom go to the hospital in this century without a lot of coaxing, let me tell you.

There are gaps in coverage which might well be filled in for a great many people, but that is quite different from adding new out-patient benefits just to use up the union health fund, or to shelter a little more income from the Internal Revenue Service, or to impose your own ideas of the best way someone else should spend his disposable income.

The Assignment of Benefits

Having looked at how fourth-parties distort the third-party mechanism, let us look at assignment of benefits, wherein the third party tries to get the patient out of its hair.

'Assignment' is an insurance term for the process by which the beneficiary of a policy (i.e., the patient) assigns the benefit (payment of the money) to the provider of care (i.e., the hospital or doctor). If payment is to flow directly from insurance company to hospital, the patient must execute an assignment authorization form. After all, the insurance contract is between the insurance company and the patient.

With assignment, there are conveniences to the patient in not having to bother with bills, payment and reimbursement, and conveniences to the hospital in being paid more quickly. On the other hand, if assignment becomes widespread, all three parties in the arrangement begin to forget their basic obligations. For the patient, the transaction becomes invisible; moral hazard is increased.

Four arguments are made for assignment of benefits. The first is a very superficial cost analysis of the clerical time spent on each paper; it is probably true that claims prepared by a doctor's secretary are more complete and legible than the tremulous efforts of grandmothers. Another is that assignment helps untangle the financial problems which develop when a patient dies or becomes incompetent. Thirdly, the system does give the insurance company some power to satisfy itself that moral hazard has not taken the form of inaccurate or excessive fees. If the provider and insurance company claims department are in direct business communication with each other, the very fact of communication provides a vehicle for asking questions which would be blocked by the interposition of the patient. Finally, the unions and employers, who usually organize insured groups, are relieved of the cost and bother of dealing with complaints or requests for assistance. They like the image of worry-free insurance.

The negative side of assigned claims is considerable. The insurance claims department is put to the added cost and delay of maintaining both a reference file of beneficiaries and a reference file of providers. The problem of maintaining a provider file is greatly magnified when there are multiple providers for each illness (one or more doctors, the hospital, possibly a laboratory, a radiologist component of an X-ray, pharmacy, surgical supplies, etc., etc.) The multiplication of providers also multiplies the complexity of dealing with a central problem for claims agents: duplicate claims. When a carrier is dealing with fifty- to seventy-thousand claims a day, he has a major technical problem of detecting double billing. If he pays too quickly, the double payment is issued and must be recaptured. If he pays too slowly, the provider assumes the claim is lost, and submits a second one. Generally, it saves money in the long run to pay quickly ("the cheapest claim is the claim you pay") because incitement of the claimant to repeat billing can paralyze a high volume payment operation. If such duplicate claims are filtered out by the patient, there is much less duplicate bill problem. All of this supports the firm opinion among many claims agents that assignment imposes a higher total claims processing cost than would be present in direct beneficiary reimbursement. Naturally, the advantages vary somewhat according to the type of claim.

Also, there is a little matter delicately referred to as "program integrity." If a patient submits a receipted bill as part of his claim, there is good reason to suppose that the service was actually rendered. When the claim goes directly from provider to reimbursement agent, there arises a need to perform investigation or spot checks, the need to require additional collateral documentation, and the establishment of a costly department of program integrity. Friction and hassle lead to bad public image for government programs, or loss of business for insurance companies. Result: pressure on the claims department not to be so fussy.

A convincing argument therefore exists that most health insurance carriers and intermediaries are better off if assignment of benefits is kept to a minimum. In an era of tight money and high interest rates, a new consideration appears. The creditors want to be paid quickly, the debtors are in no hurry. Your payables are my receivables. Whenever there is the slightest delay in the transaction, someone has to borrow money. If a hospital has to borrow money, the interest cost is reimbursable, and the cost-reimbursement agency or insuror has to pay the interest cost. There is good reason to curtail assignment of benefits almost altogether, as will be suggested in a later chapter.

Self-Insurance

One of the most dramatic changes in health insurance in recent years has been the discovery that it is highly advantageous to both company and customer if the insurance company stops writing (that is, underwriting) health insurance entirely. The process is known as self-insurance, but it seems scarcely different from real insurance to the customer except for the important point that it is usually cheaper.

To help understand self-insurance, here is a short course in the insurance business, which can be divided into four areas:

1. Sales, marketing, and premium collection.
2. Risk assessment and premium setting.
3. Investment portfolio management (of the premium money).
4. Claims payment.

Observers of the health insurance market began to see that the great bulk of health insurance was being marketed to employer-employee groups. Such groups were then "experience-rated," which is to say their premium was based on the previous year's experience for the group rather than on the performance of the insurance company's whole book of business. It next became apparent to very large employers that there was very little year-to-year variation in the premiums, except for inflation. In other words, there was very little risk; and since there was little risk, there was little need to pay the insurance company to protect against risk.

Furthermore, there was no marketing cost, and very little sense to going through the motions of premium collection. What would the insurance company charge *just to pay the claims out of the company bank account*? For their part, insurance companies did not regard health insurance as particularly profitable, were apprehensive that some sort of nationalization of health insurance was coming, and were pretty fed up with being squeezed each year between inflation and the need to persuade insurance commissioners to permit premium increases. So, many insurance companies were willing to administer to employee group health plans for a fixed percentage of the transactions. During periods of inflation and high interest rates, as it happens, the administration fee is about equal to the interest on the premium money (which remains with the company until needed). A large corporation may thus reduce the cost of its fringe benefit to an absolute minimum, retain professional management of its claims administration, eliminate most of the need for portfolio management, and still remain in a position to take bids from competitive insurance companies for better or cheaper claims administration. The claims administrator, on the other hand, has a steady business of predictable profitability, needs no longer be embarrassed by portfolio losses in the bond market, and can ignore the insurance commissioner. Instead of profits one year and losses the next, the insurance companies enjoy a moderate, steady income.

What so far has been described is an approach which has been widely adopted by large corporations with thousands of employees. Smaller groups have special problems, and there are certain extra risks which have to be addressed. The first risk is that an epidemic, an act of God, or the law of averages will cause the small group to incur an unsupportable medical expense in one year. Solution: purchase reinsurance against catastrophes.

A second problem for small self-insurance groups may be that their management is unwilling to undertake the investment burden because of inexperience, preoccupation with other things, or the inability to achieve predictable investment results with small sums. However, professional investment with guaranteed returns is available.

So, at some additional cost of reinsurance and investment guarantee, small groups are able to enjoy the benefits of self-insurance just as though they were major national corporations. The extra costs are sometimes absorbed by two interesting quirks—relief from nongroup subsidy, and relief from teaching hospital subsidy.

In the first place, group subscribers are sometimes forced by the insurance commissioner to inflate their premiums in order to permit the insurance company to undercharge the individual non-group subscribers to the plan. Small groups are usually less alert and less powerful than large groups, so their premiums are particularly affected. The small group thus may find it has a differential cost disadvantage, the elimination of which makes up for some of the extra costs of self-insurance.

Some small groups may also find that most of their members go to small suburban or other nonteaching hospitals, where the charges are considerably less than those of teaching hospitals, and the contractual discounts (see "A Primer From The Trustees") are less. Since policies which offer service benefits are overcharging the patient who goes to a non-teaching hospital in order to subsidize the patient who goes to a teaching hospital, it may pay some groups to escape the "community-rated" premium structure. Community rating, the opposite of experience rating, increases the moral hazard. It would mean that nothing you could do about your costs would reduce your premium. While these two features of small groups are subject to great individual variation, the very considerable recent growth of self-insurance almost certainly means it results in appreciable savings to many customers. If tight money and high interest rates continue, the cash flow issue may seem even more important to management than minor cost considerations.

It would appear that small-group self-insurance is making considerable inroads, so it would be well to ponder the consequences of a possible massive shift in that direction. It is clear that an immediate effect of "skimming off the cream" (or releasing the victim from bondage) would be an increase in the premiums for the nongroup subscribers (or a return to proper level, as you please). It further seems likely that such a trend in insurance will have the effect of encouraging patients to seek lower-cost (usually suburban) hospitals instead of higher-cost (usually center-city, teaching) hospitals.

It would be hard to identify anyone who would be indifferent to the possibility that a stampede to group self-insurance might set off an upward spiral of nongroup premiums. The Blue plans might well be transformed into assigned-risk pools so rapidly that they could not survive. (There are anti-trust implications to assigned-risk pools between competing insurance companies. Even if the companies were willing to take this step, it might be hampered by the anti-trust issue.) The consequence of anything approaching such developments would surely be political interference, so group self-insurance must pass its political test before it can be considered a permanent factor of consequence.

15

Sticky Wicket

Mr. Spalding was thirty-six years old, his cousin Mr. Wallis was nearly seventy. The vagaries of inherited estates plus the tricky alliances of family politics had resulted in the younger man being president of the family glue business, while the older man was merely treasurer. Both of them enjoyed musty old offices, with inherited roll top desks. Mr. Wallis actually used his roll top, which suited him very well after forty years. Mr. Spalding mostly used his desk as a conversation piece for visitors, and a place to put his Hasty Pudding bowl. He did his work at a table in the center of the room which his secretary kept completely bare except for the single paper Mr. Spalding happened to be reading or signing. Mr. Wallis had hung some Birch and Krimmel engravings, whereas Mr. Spalding went in for horsey pictures. Just over the roll top were two very small snapshots. One of them showed him on a horse, much younger, in the uniform of the City Troop. Beside it was a picture of his father, shaking hands with the Queen of England.

The two had been talking for an hour, and had made up their minds about a personnel matter. "Let's call in Allan and let him listen," said Mr. Spalding. "He's your grandson and I know you can fill him in later, but he ought to get a chance to hear it discussed. And ask Edith to tell O'Toole that we're ready for him."

Mr. Wallis nodded. "Do you want to go over to O'Toole's office? It's always a courteous thing to go to a man's office when you have bad news for him."

"What's so bad about it? Anyway, I can't stand that gaudy bordello that he uses for an office."

"Well," said the older man, "you are telling him to change a basic policy in his department. You know he doesn't want to, and you know you are going to make him do it anyway. That's bad news for most of us egotists. But no matter He can hear it in this office."

Almost instantly, Mr. O'Toole, the personnel manager of the glue company, appeared. All smiles, and suntan from his cabin cruiser. It took a few minutes more for young Allan Wallis to appear, since he had tried to finish up with the employee who had been talking to him when the presidential summons arrived, whereas Mr. O'Toole had simply broken off and left. Each knew it of the other. One scorned nepotism, and the other disdained sychophancy.

As the meeting settled down, Mr. Wallis and his grandson quietly faded into the wallpaper. The conversation was to be between their cousin and his hatchet man, and it was best not to get too close.

"Mr. O'Toole, Mr. Wallis and I have been looking over the savings you achieved for us by dropping the employee group health insurance and going self-insured. That's really pretty neat."

At this, Mr. O'Toole breathed a sigh of relief. So that was it. Maybe a raise. He asked me to his office, so I might have known it was good news. Obviously, self-insured employee health benefits were the way to go.

"Thanks, Mr. Spalding. It has worked rather well. I picked up the idea at the Glue Manufacturers Association meeting in San Diego last year. Big old wooden hotel on the beach. They say the Duke of Windsor first met Wally there in the bar." Unseen by O'Toole, Mr. Wallis's eyes narrowed slightly.

Spalding continued, "Yes, you're giving us quite an education. The insurance carrier we used to have would adjust each year's premium to pay for the previous year's experience. Well, we might just as well have kept the premium money and earned interest on it. Mr. Wallis, senior, is able to get us 10 percent on the premium money in a money market fund. So, if we pay half of that to an insurance carrier to handle bookkeeping, we've just saved 5 percent of health costs, which are 10 percent of employee costs. So our company's margin just widened. Very good."

"As a matter of fact," murmured the senior Mr. Wallis, "I've had to pay 14 percent interest to the bank on our credit line lately to finance inventory. So it's better for us just to reduce our line of credit than to try to draw interest on the cash."

Mr. Spalding leaned forward to recapture attention. "So now quite obviously, there are some internal company management rearrangements which have to be made." Mr. O'Toole's back stiffened. Watch out; something's up. What was that kid doing here at this meeting? My God, they're going to give him my job. Mr. Spalding's voice, now rather remote from his body, resumed.

"So, you see, we are now in a position to close the medical department."

Mr. O'Toole, his mind violently thrashing to imagine what conspiracy was being plotted, was completely taken aback. "I'm sorry, but I don't understand at all."

Spalding smiled in a friendly way and continued, "As you have heard me say before, my family has never liked the idea of requiring a physical examination on a prospective new employee before we hired him. It tends to mean that a sick person can't get a job." Mr. O'Toole ruffled up. "Mr. Spalding, when I took this job I was promised a free hand. And when I took this job, the employee ranks were filled with broken-down parasites on the payroll. A sick employee is an expensive employee. The pre-employment physical is a vital component of modern personnel management." Wallis senior had told Spalding to expect something like this, and the coach was curious to see how his player handled it.

Spalding got up, went to the door, and asked Edith if she would bring in a pot of coffee for the meeting. In coming back to his chair, he walked behind O'Toole, who twisted uncomfortably to watch him. "Yes," he said, "things change, even in the glue business. People come and go. But the Spalding Glue Company has been a family business for ninety-six years. Ten years ago there were six other family glue businesses in this town, but now there is only one. Robinson was bought out by the Texas Company, Hoffman is part of Sears Roebuck, and the others went broke. Only Spalding is left as a family business, and we do owe a lot to you for keeping it that way. But there really is no sense in our having a family business unless we can run it like a family. We do not like easing people out of a job because they are sick. We think we can afford not to do it. And we're not going to do it."

O'Toole fought for time. Perhaps he should throw his job in their faces, but he suspected that there were more cards to be turned over. He couldn't imagine they would suddenly make an issue of this stupid thing unless they had something else in mind. If they had already decided to give his job to that kid, he would be in a better bargaining position if he hadn't been maneuvered into quitting. Let's see. One more year for pension vesting, four more for early retirement. After a brief moment, he asked, "What suddenly brought this up, anyway?"

"Mostly, I have been looking over the hospital bills we have been paying for our employees. Now that we pay them ourselves instead of having them filter through an insurance premium, they don't seem so unreasonable. The prices those hospitals charge are pretty high, but I'm on the board of the hospital near my place in the country, and they have their problems. Those prices aren't going down. And if the doctor's fees are high, well, we would be doing our medical director a favor by firing him and forcing him to go into practice."

"What about the annual executive physicals?" asked O'Toole, who really couldn't understand what this was all about, and was probing.

"As a matter of fact, Mr. Wallis discovered an interesting thing about that over at the Pickwick Club. Tell him, Bruce."

The company treasurer answered, "As you know, there's a doctor who sits at our table regularly. Has some kind of a damned beeper that goes off during lunch, but he's otherwise all right. I asked him what it would cost to get a complete checkup in his office, or one like it. He said about a hundred dollars.

"Well, I didn't say this to him, but those executive examination clinics charge twice that. So it looks to me as though having our medical director do the exams isn't the bargain we though it was—it's just a bargain compared with the clinics. Personally, I'm in favor of giving the employee the money and letting him pick his own doctor."

"But, Mr. Wallis, then he would have to pay for it in after-tax dollars," protested O'Toole.

"Maybe so, but it rubs me the wrong way to pay double for something just to get a 50 percent tax discount. The thing that ought to be bothering us is the way our executives get so dependent on the company that they don't know any doctors when they wake up with a heart attack."

O'Toole did not intend to yield. This was his field of work, and he knew it thoroughly. "It can sometimes be vital to know about an employee's health. When you are reviewing him for possible promotion."

At this, Spalding intervened. "Now, just a damned minute. This is the first time I ever even heard such an idea. If we have any such policy, please consider it reversed as of this moment. Or maybe I didn't hear you right."

Before O'Toole could react to this novel development, Spalding resumed. "And if, by any conceivable chance, we should find that we have to snoop into our employee's private lives to keep the company from bankruptcy, the personnel records are good enough. We know how many days they were sick, we know how much they cost us. We know it for each one, and we can lump it together by department or split it up by sex and age. Personally, I hope I never see the day when we have to do that sort of stuff to be able to compete in the glue business. But if we ever do have to face the issue, we can face it then."

O'Toole was absolutely certain there was more to this than he had heard, and he wasn't going to say anything definite until he learned what it was. "You know," he started tentatively, "General Motors sends a bigger check to Blue Cross than it does to US Steel."

"Yes, I heard that fellow from GM say so at the Chamber of Commerce. But I imagine they send lots of checks to Inland Steel and Bethlehem Steel."

"And the Japanese steel companies," jabbed O'Toole.

"Fair enough. Fair enough," said the senior Wallis, rising from his chair. "With your new increase in salary, Mr. O'Toole, perhaps you can visit Japan to see the modern industrial miracle."

After the briefest of startled pauses, O'Toole started laughing. "So that's it. I get a raise and you guys are trying to enjoy yourselves when you give it to me. That's pretty good. That's rich."

Young Spalding rose, and showed O'Toole to the door with his hand on his shoulder. "Sure. Ten percent and fringes. I'll write you a memo this afternoon." O'Toole was two steps out the door. "And by the way." O'Toole stopped and turned to hear Mr. Spalding's final pleasantry. "You write me a memo today about how you are doing to implement that new medical policy."

16

The New Poor: Money Isn't Everything

A century ago, it was reasonable to say that everyone was rich, poor, or middle class, and that medical care was determined by social position. We continue to employ the rhetoric of social class in describing medical care, but a century of social change and social legislation has made the old slogans obsolete. As a general rule, the 1965 Medicaid and Medicare acts made it unnecessary for anyone to alter or lower his standards of medical care for reasons of money, and they also started the slower process of upgrading the quality of care received by those who had been indigent before the social legislation was passed. Growls began to emerge from the middle class that they were more pinched by medical expenses than they would be if they were poor, and the upwardly mobile on the way from lower to middle class discovered that when things stop being free, you have to pay for them.

Exceptions and variations do exist. While Medicare is a national program, Medicaid is a system of federal matching money, available to states which established federally approved programs. All states except Arizona developed such programs, but they varied greatly in their generosity and coverage. Some states held back on implementing Medicaid programs, and only grudgingly later liberalized the bare minimum. Other states, like California and New York, enthusiastically extended generous maximum benefits as soon as the federal matching money became available, but the costs soon became so high that they have had to suffer the unpopularity of reducing and restricting the benefits. Because no one wishes to attract out-of-state welfare recipients to a generous welfare program, residency and other eligibility requirements are almost universally very difficult. Many states have had political difficulty dealing with problems which have a moral taint, like spending state tax revenues to pay for abortions, care for illegitimate children, or treatment of venereal disease, alcoholism, or drug addiction. Some of the state programs have probably been poorly administered, but it is difficult to sort out the politically motivated attacks from objective appraisals. Fraud and abuse may possibly exist, although sensationalism must be discounted, especially before an election.

But for all the spottiness which may exist in the Medicaid programs, it remains essentially true that the cost of acute medical care for those of low income has been accepted by Medicaid, and there is no financial reason why the care should be inferior. Nevertheless, a large subculture of medically underserved continues to exist. Just to list typical underserved groups may assist in the understanding of the problem:

- Recent legal immigrants (i.e., boat people, etc.)
- Illegal immigrants (i.e., wetbacks, etc.)
- Skid row alcoholics
- Drug addicts
- Younger vagrants, such as "hippies"
- Gypsies
- Mentally retarded (especially after parents die)
- Semisenile older vagrants
- Criminal elements, prostitutes, gamblers
- Prison inmates
- Marginally competent psychotics
- Extreme neurotic recluses
- Lifetime ghetto residents

All of the members of the above list might well be completely covered by Medicaid, Medicare, or other financial protection but the quality of their medical care could still be very substandard. Probably is, in fact. The unifying characteristic of those people is not that they are poor (although they may be); it is that they are not full members of our culture. It is extraordinary how often they change their residence, for instance. As dissatisfied with their environment as the environment is dissatisfied with them, they wander. The national census has a repeated problem accounting for the disappearance of large numbers of black males between the ages of 17 and 40. They rejoin society in middle age, but they vanish for a time. One can hope that education and social programs will eventually conquer this problem; but the problem of the abandoned elderly is just beginning and will inevitably grow much worse.

The most visible familiar representative of the new poor is the shopping-bag lady. No doubt you have seen her on the busy street corner, and if you have a regular schedule it will strike you that she has one, too. Usually on the move, she is at the same place at the same time every day. You may have smelled her, too; the strong odor of stale urine often characteristic of subway stations.

Perhaps your city has a skid row which you pass on your way to your own world. Many of its sad derelicts are alcoholics and drug addicts, but many are merely grown-up mentally retarded children, or grown-up mentally disturbed children. Almost all are harmless victims, even when they act as petty predators on each other. They are seldom a match for the most defenseless of comfortable citizens.

In 1750, Benjamin Franklin composed a petition for the Provincial Legislature of Pennsylvania, and obtained the signatures of thirty-three prominent citizens. Although the petition was in his own handwriting, for some reason he did not sign it.

> The Petition of sundry Inhabitants of the said Province humbly sheweth,
> *That* with the numbers of People, the number of Lunaticks or Persons distempered in Mind and deprived of their rational Faculties, both greatly increased in this Province.
> *That* some of them going at large are a Terror to their Neighbors, who are daily apprehensive of the Violence they may commit: And others are continually wasting their Substance, to the great Injury of themselves and Families, ill disposed Persons wickedly taking advantage of their unhappy Condition, and drawing them into unreasonable Bargains.
> *That* few or none of them are sensible of their Condition, as to submit voluntarily to the Treatment their respective Cases require, and therefore continue in the same deplorable State during their Lives . . . .
> *Your* Petitioners beg leave farther to represent,
> *That* the good Laws of the Province have made many compassionate and charitable Provisions for the relief of the Poor, yet something farther seems wanting in favor of such, whose Poverty is made more miserable by the additional Weight of grievous Disease . . . .
> *The* kind Care our Assemblies have heretofore taken for the Relief of sick and distempered Strangers, by providing a Place for their Reception and

Accommodation, leaves us no room to doubt their showing an equal tender Concern for the Inhabitants. And we hope they will be of opinion with us, that a small Provincial Hospital erected and put under proper Regulations, in the care of Persons to be appointed by this House, or otherwise as they think meet, with Power to receive and apply the charitable Benefactions of good People towards enlarging and supporting the same, and some other Provision in a Law for the Purposes above mentioned, will be a good Work, acceptable to God and to all the good People they present.

We therefore recommend the premises to their serious Consideration.

Aside from the quaintness of the language, Mr. Franklin's petition would seem to be as pertinent today as it was two hundred years ago. The hospital he suggested was built, and many others, too. Why haven't things changed?

It is true that many well-informed experts in the fields of mental retardation and mental disorder feel that "snake-pit" state-run mental hospitals did a disservice. They were often human warehouses which kept the social problems out of sight and out of mind. Powerful mood-altering drugs have now made it possible for many former inmates to function adequately in society. And it is true that society should help these people live their lives in freedom, searching for what crumbs of happiness they can find, wherever that is practical.

At the same time, we must be wary of self-serving by state government. General prosperity and full employment have made custodial care in institutions crushingly expensive. However capital-intensive we may make our institutions, custodial care is still a very labor-intensive system. The states have only a limited amount of money to spend on social services, and "reintegrating" the new poor "into society" is one way to make funds available for higher priorities. Looking ahead, the aging of the population is inevitably destined to enlarge the pool of mentally enfeebled new poor. What we are going to do about it isn't clear.

Special Problems of the Poor

It seems to me that the new way to address the medical problems of the poor is to recognize that poorness is no longer the central medical issue with the poor. Indeed, a medical problem is often the cause of the poorness, particularly in the case of diseases affecting the brain like schizophrenia, alcoholism, drug addiction, mental retardation, senility. The causes of medical indigency are so unrelated to each other that the best approach would probably be to chip away at the solvable problems with a wide variety of special programs. These people, in other words, would be better treated as any one of twenty different problems, than lumped together under the single heading of poverty. Taking that approach, there is less chance that we will impose distortions on the mainstream of health care, where maximum use of self-help and market incentives works best. When a class of people lies clearly outside the marketplace, its special nonmarket characteristics must be accomodated.

In addition to being poor, and largely outside the medical market economy, these people have created three special problems for the health care system. It is important that we recognize the problems inherent in free drug programs, low fixed-fee schedules, and the abuse of hospital emergency departments. We begin with the subject of Medicaid Mills.

Shared Health Facilities

Newspapers coined the term "Medicaid Mills" for certain high-volume, low-prestige medical offices which were given great notoriety by the congressional hearings chaired by Representative Moss of California. Mr. Moss had actually put on a dirty shirt, posed as a Medicaid recipient, and presented himself for care in some ghetto clinics. He was clearly upset with what seemed to be evidence of fraud and abuse, and even more upset with the lack of suitable laws or enforcement efforts by government supervisory agencies. The ultimate outcome of this notoriety was the Medicare and Medicaid Fraud and Abuse Act, sponsored by Representative Rostenkowski of Illinois.

Representative Rostenkowski's committee had the difficult task of defining the abuse which was to be curtailed, and to frame legislation which would curtail abusive practices, without also hampering legitimate professional latitude or totally depriving ghetto areas of any medical care at all. The problem was considerably hampered by the fact that the federal Medicaid matching money which Congress had a right to regulate was dispensed by the states through forty-nine different programs. Since many of the issues are covert, it is difficult to get the facts on which to base conclusions, even in your own neighborhood.

However, it is pretty clear that ghetto patients only have a realistic choice between care at a hospital out-patient clinic, and care at what is now, for better or worse, called a Medicaid Mill.

Since out-patient clinics have been hopelessly stigmatized by ghetto patients as symbols of degrading wooden-bench charity, patients mostly refuse to go there. Even if they didn't have to wait so long, even if the "medical students in white coats" were to be replaced by mature physicians in business suits, even if the waiting rooms were to have Swedish modern furniture and piped-in music, it still wouldn't do. People in the ghetto are influenced by one standard. It has to be like what television tells them is the way medicine is practiced in the suburbs. Neither is the out-patient clinic welcome to the hospital, which loses money on it. Physicians are hard to find to staff it because most prefer a suburban career model or an in-patient consultant model. Most hospitals either have closed their clinics for lack of clients, or else they clearly wish they could close them. Finally, the hospital clinic is not financially attractive for the fiscal agency. For a variety of reasons, and in spite of efforts to shift indirect costs to the in-patient area, clinic visits cost almost twice as much as gold-coast suburban office visits.

Meanwhile, a basic obstacle remains: Medical practice in ghetto areas is usually distressing to middle-class providers of care, generally lacking in glamour for employees, and often physically unsafe. If practitioners in these areas are further stigmatized with the term "Medicaid Mill," the difficulty of attracting practitioners to the area is only exacerbated further. If ghetto areas are to receive medical care equal to that in the suburbs, differential incentives obviously must be created. While a few states like California and New York briefly and temporarily provided reasonable reimbursement for Medicaid recipients, even these states have retreated back into the fiscal stringency of the low-fee schedule, limited-number-of-visits-per-month, restricted-use-of-ancillary-services sort, which most of the other states had never relaxed. It seems inevitable that ghetto patients will be permanently condemmed to substandard care unless either other incentives are devised, or the financial incentive is revived.

Other incentives have been hard to improvise. Mexico requires every medical graduate whose education had been paid for by the government to spend some time after graduation in underserved areas, and there have been proposals to bring this system north of the Rio Grande. The Indian Health Service, run by the United States Public Health Service, has been suggested as a possible model, but both of these systems have their problems, and, in any event, do not look enough like suburban medicine to be certain of patient acceptance. Various experimental clinics funded by the government and run by neighborhood groups have generally proved to be extremely expensive, occasionally blemished by financial scandal, and not better accepted by ghetto residents than hospital out-patient clinics. An occasional dedicated medical missionary has translated the zeal and methods of Albert Schweitzer to the urban jungle, but the infrequency of such projects demonstrates the paucity of Dr. Livingstons, we presume. After all, one must also contend with the feelings of Mrs. Schweitzer and Mrs. Livingston, who generally do not enjoy the experience of worrying about periodic muggings of their husbands.

So, what are Medicaid Mills all about, anyway? In the first place, a majority of their physicians are young, and fairly well-trained. Most of them work part-time and plan to stay in the ghetto only until their second office in the suburbs can support them. The Moss hearings stimulated some studies of the quality of care delivered, and the New York Professional Standards Review Organization was unable to demonstrate that the quality of care was inferior to that provided by the out-patient clinics of some prestigious New York teaching hospitals. The fraud and abuse investigative agency known as the Office of Program Integrity has rarely been able to demonstrate kick-backs, fraudulent claims, or other signs of passing money illegally. So what was all this fuss about Medicaid Mills?

Well, in the first place, it is difficult to answer the claim that the Moss hearings and the Rostenkowski law put a stop to fraudulent practices which flourished formerly; there is now no way to know. Secondly, occasional cases continue to hit the headlines of ghetto practitioners who are found to be illicitly supplying what is known as the "drug scene." And finally, the enormous volume of reported office visits in a limited time period continues to suggest on the surface that such brief visits might not have been of high quality.

In discussing this problem with a respected physician friend of mine, he remarked, "I once practiced in a Medicaid Mill. It was called the United States Air Force base dispensary. We saw eighty patients a day, and we didn't do so badly by them. We even kept good records, although of course we never looked at them. You do what you can, when you have to." Anyone who has looked at military records knows that they are so voluminous that no one could use them. It is far easier to ask the patient to return frequently in order to keep his problem fresh in mind until the problem is settled. The military and the welfare agencies require extensive records, but handwriting is not the time-consuming part. Reading it is what takes time. If the problem gets too complicated, there is a strong incentive to refer the patient to a hospital, and let someone else sort out the history. If the problem isn't quite bad enough for that, it is possible to have the patient keep returning until you get it straight; but reading records is out.

Now, if the Medicaid Mills represent part-time hard work in a somewhat dangerous neighborhood by young doctors getting started, the process requires a permanent owner-operator to be efficient and maintain continuity for the "practice." This individual usually is the landlord, although he may also run the drug-store, laboratory, surgical supply and appliance store, or other associated activity. The arrangement was called a Shared Health Facility by Rostenkowski law, and its operation was severely constrained. Since hospitals meet just about every point of the definition of an SHF, they were specifically exempted. The operator-owner of an SHF does a great many things to maintain his operation, which also have parallels in hospitals.

He has to get replacements for the physicians as they pull out. One of the common inducements is to lower the rent or even forgive it for a period, a practice that is not exactly unknown when a hospital is trying to induce a busy practitioner to join the hospital and fill the beds. The operator provides all the start-up arrangements and equipment; the new doctor walks into a going operation from the very first day. The operator makes it his business to know all of the constraints and loopholes of the local Medicaid law, and he is often willing to perform services of a business nature that he has learned the young doctors would be inexperienced or even squeamish about. The shifting of overhead costs is within his ability as a landlord. Services like sigmoidoscopy can be suggested as a form of subsidy for inadequate fees in other areas. Consultants can be suggested to a newcomer physician, who has an immediate need for consultants and has no time to evaluate local quality.

All of this could be defended as spontaneous accommodation to the special needs of the urban ghetto, and it can be argued that effective legislation to curtail abuse would be lacking constitutional even-handedness unless it also greatly disrupted normal practices in high prestige hospitals and medical practices. But one finds that such arguments are somehow unconvincing. One wishes all of this were not happening, and one wishes for a better system.

One has the feeling that there may be more revelations about the background of the operators of shared medical facilities, or the nature of their procedures, so that it is uncomfortable to be in the position of defending them. But there is absolutely no denying the fact that they are popular with their patients. Why else would they be called Mills?

Free Prescriptions

It does not suffice to pay for an indigent patient's visit to a doctor if the patient cannot then afford to buy his medicine. So free prescription programs are very common in Medicaid programs, but they are the occasion of some of the worst abuse. Some of those little capsules may cost a dollar apiece to someone who needs them, and may be as valuable as life itself; but to the Medicaid patient they are free. So wasteful usage occurs, getting a little extra for your friends is a temptation, and getting some extra pills to sell on the street is not unknown.

Let's keep the problem in perspective. Physician panels for review of computer summaries of Medicaid prescriptions find that the great majority, say 95 percent, of patients and prescriptions seem to reflect appropriate usage patterns. But the programs include millions of recipients, and millions of prescriptions. The amount of tranquilizers consumed by some recipients can be astonishing, and the doctor can never be certain when the patient is really swallowing the pills or giving them to others. The frequency with which falsified names and medical assistance cards turn up suggests that underworld activity is distinctly possible. A few people are apparently creating a lot of abuse.

Such evidence of abuse inevitably leads to regulatory reaction.

Only so many pills may be prescribed at any one time. Only so many refills are permitted. Patients with high usage are restricted to a single doctor and a single pharmacy. Permissable tranquilizers are limited to one or two cheap ones. Unannounced audits are performed in drugstores. Agents visit the patient at home to make inquiries.

Medical Assistance programs really should search for some cash substitutes for free prescriptions, but the problem of tranquilizer abuse probably does require regulation to prevent free drug programs from corrupting our whole society. A moral of this mess is this: Don't extend prepaid drug programs to people who can afford to buy their drugs. There is probably no escape from some free drugs for the indigents, but it's bad news for anybody else, believe me.

Growing Emergency

There are two traditions for hospital emergency rooms. The newer tradition is the one displayed on television, with excitement, helicopters, catastrophes, narrow escapes, lots of flashing lights, and lots of blood. The older tradition is for hospital emergency departments to serve as family doctor for the poor. The new tradition is sometimes seen in the suburbs and rural hospitals, although such accident rooms are mainly quiet and lonesome during the intervals between the arrivals of state policemen with the victims of highway smash-ups. A great deal of expensive standby equipment and personnel stands idle much of the time, resembling very much the scene in firehouses. When we drive on interstate highways we like to think there is a well-equipped and staffed emergency facility not too far from anywhere, and keeping it in readiness costs a lot. We don't care, we want it available.

If your accident should occur close to a large urban hospital, however, you will find the situation is different. The emergency room will have a large waiting room, and it will usually be full. The waiting clients will probably have a seamy look about them. Some of them may just be there to get warm, some of them look half-dead.

Long ago, the medical system developed a tradition of treating the episodic illnesses of the poor in the accident room. Acute trauma is understood to require constant standby, and acute trauma is more often a nosebleed, a sprained ankle, or a small cut than it is a gunshot wound or auto smashup. Indeed, in the city, vehicle velocity is slower, so even the auto injuries are less spectacular. Knife wounds, broken jaws, and broken knuckles are more typical. But even these acute injuries are diluted by a host of people with colds, venereal disease, belly aches, and nervous complaints. Innumerable head nurses have scolded patients for bringing minor complaints to an overcongested emergency department, but the sheepish look tells all. The problem seemed important at the time.

Because the emergency department cannot take a chance on turning away anyone for fear he drop dead, the tradition of bad debts is also associated with these facilities. It is understandable that people in an emergency may forget their insurance card or wallet. It is less understandable that they occasionally give a false address or a fictitious name. Sometimes the local community or state government or United Fund will cover such bad debts; but often not. Not only may the charge for the visit be lost, but there are additional uncollectible charges for the 4.94 units of laboratory work and 0.45 X-ray procedures which were associated last year nationally with the average emergency room visit. The hospital financial department is therefore not exactly greedy to encourage more accident room visits. In addition, it is said that almost half of all malpractice suits against hospitals begin in the accident room. Many hospitals have annual malpractice premiums in excess of a million dollars. It would be tempting to cut that cost in half by eliminating the emergency room entirely.

But our present concern is with the poor, many of whom regard the accident room as their doctor. Why isn't this a solution to care in the ghetto? Primarily, it is an unsatisfactory stop-gap because it doesn't, and can't, provide continuity of care. If your nosebleed is a one-time thing, the accident room will stop it for you. But if your nosebleed comes from high blood pressure, they cannot permit you to keep coming back to have it treated. If you have a heart attack, they can admit you to the hospital; but when you leave the hospital you can't keep coming back to the accident room for continuing care. They even have a problem taking out the stitches after you have had your cut sewed up. They may write voluminous notes about your problem, but they mostly do it for legal protection. If you come back later, the record of your previous visit is usually too hard to find to bother looking for.

Continuity of care requires stability and good memories. The doctor knows that his notes become useless if they are voluminous; he writes his own short-hand to aid his memory. The patient's memory is essential, too. He relates his other problems, and reminds the doctor what has taken place. A continuing dialogue is needed. When the patient suffers from mental incapacity, or when he never sees two doctors twice in a row, or when he stays away for long periods of time, voluminous records become necessary. The problems of ghetto medicine revolve around all of the factors which make it difficult to maintain continuity of care, and neither bulky records nor hospital accident rooms are the proper solution, even if costs were favorable. Unfortunately, the average cost of an emergency room visit was nationally reported by the Hospital Activity Summary in 1978 to be $38.64. Look at what happened to accident room visits in the 242 hospitals of Pennsylvania in the past 5 years:

1972	3,501,170
1973	3,771,359
1974	4,241,973
1975	4,268,824
1976	4,545,559
1977	4,544,960

At a time when days-of-care rendered in these hospitals only increased 2 percent, and when there is no reason to suppose the number of emergencies changed, the number of visits increased by a million a year. It may be unfair to say that the extra visits cost $38 million in one state per year. But surely it is correct to say it is an unfortunate trend for accident room visits to increase 25 percent in five years when the facility is both unsatisfactory for continuing care as well as fiercely expensive. And it clogs up the real emergency system, so that you and I aren't certain of immediate attention when we have our turnpike accident.

One has to develop the resigned view that the solution to the problem of providing medical care to the poor is going to come slowly, and its future direction will depend on massive societal forces beyond the control of the medical system. If the elderly decide to migrate to the suburbs, a suburban solution will evolve. If they continue their historical pattern of moving from center city more slowly than younger people, the problem will require an inner-city solution. If we develop a system of day-care centers for the elderly as they have done in Finland, medical care will probably take place in these centers. If we have a major depression, or a war, or accelerated inflation, something else will happen. The purpose of this chapter is not to define how to solve the monumental problem of the medically underserved. It is to suggest that merely broadening health insurance coverage is a long way from what will ultimately put things right.

17

Guardians of the Poor

"It's my deal. We'll just ruffle up the tickets and have a little seven-card stud, nothing wild. Ante up two of those blue ones." The speaker, Big Bill O'Toole, a forty-year-old man in shirt sleeves, was minority leader of the House of Burgesses of the state legislature. At the moment, in a hotel room ten blocks from the capital, late at night, he was deeply into the regular dealer's-choice meeting of a friendly group of legislative poker players. They were all family men, stranded in hotel rooms three or four days a week while the legislature met. They were surprisingly young, since state politics is a stepping-stone to other things, and it gets boring after a few years if you don't move up. Nights in a hotel room are the worst part of it. The senior of the group was a former legislator who had been given a job in the Health and Welfare Department, and had continued to remain a member of the poker group after his wife died: Jim Hostetter.

Big Bill O'Toole continued the chatter. "All right, you've all got your down cards. Put up your antes. Come on, Lien, cover the cards with two blue chips. Don't pretend you didn't notice. You're playing with an eagle-eyed dealer who holds you to the rules."

"Speaking of rules," said an enormous former football star named Rineman, "hey, listen. We need your Rules Committee to give us an open rule on the Mental Health Bill."

"We'll see, we'll see," smiled O'Toole over his tightly clenched cigar. The Rules Committee enjoyed its mysterious powers, and seldom announced its intentions in advance.

"Hey, look, that's no way to run things. Those power-mad-ding-a-lings on your Rules Committee haven't got the faintest idea what's going on. Hey, really!"

"We'll see what we can do," nodded O'Toole. "Are you going to bet on that jack, or not?"

"Hey, you've got me so upset with your Rules Committee. I haven't had time to consider my down cards, so I pass."

"Uh huh, yeah," said someone, and the thought was mentally echoed by the rest of the players.

Mr. Hostetter thought it might be a good time to work for defeat of that bill, which would have released the institutionalized mental patients who were now in the state hospitals. "You know, that bill in its present form is just crazy. You can't take those people we have in the state hospital and turn them loose; that's absurd," he said.

"It would save lots of bucks for the state," answered O'Toole, "and the social workers tell us it's the latest trend. They have done it successfully in New York."

"Like Hell!" answered Rineman. "Hey, you know those clowns in New York are just taking some old run-down hotels off the hands of the owners at a big profit. Hey, you know it just saves them the trouble of selling those places to the fire insurance company, and they call that reintegrating the patients into the community. Hey, you know what a crock that is."

Mr. Hostetter laughed. "When you've been in the health and welfare game for a few years, you see that the pendulum just swings back and forth. We used to be battered with criticism about how it was a sin to have those insane people out in the flophouses. Get them into the hospitals where they can be treated, they said. Well, we got the hospitals built and then the same people started complaining that they were snake pits. So, now it's a sin to deprive those poor souls of normal life in the community. Five years from now we'll be hearing how shocking it is that we rank fiftieth in the nation in providing modern treatment facilities."

"Hey, yeah," said Rineman, "and what big real estate promoter has his eye on acquiring the grounds of the hospital? That's eighteen acres of pretty choice real estate."

"Damn!" shouted O'Toole. "When I'm the dealer, I never have any good cards. I'll stick, but it's just because it's my game. Damn it to hell!" The cards went round, face up, with no particular public clues. Everyone stayed with the raises, with Lien doing most of the raising.

"What are you so proud of, Lien? You must have something up your sleeve, because you don't have anything on the table."

Mr. Hostetter resumed his lobbying. "You guys are so free with money, I hope you are just as easygoing when you appropriate money for my department."

O'Toole grunted. "Look, pal, if you think I'm going to vote to raise the sales tax just to take care of your kooks, you don't know me very well. I'm planning to come back here again next year, and try to win back my money from this poker group."

"I understand," answered Hostetter, "and I felt the same way when I was in the House. But just remember the federal matching money. Every dollar you give my department brings an extra dollar into the state from Washington."

"Nuts to that stuff," answered Lien. "I'm sick and tired of being blackmailed by Washington with their conditional grants. They've got this cute trick of passing a law saying the state can only get the money if the state changes its laws. So they get around the Constitution with the blackmail approach. The Constitution clearly says the states have exclusive autonomy in anything that isn't reserved to the federal. As far as I'm concerned, the job of the federal government is to deliver the mail and defend the coasts. And come to think of it, it doesn't even do those two things very well. By the way, I raise you ten."

"I'll see you ten, although I think I'm going out of my mind with all of this chatter," said O'Toole. "Why don't you guys play cards? Unless maybe you want to introduce a constitutional amendment forbidding conditional federal grants."

Hostetter looked thoughtful. "Hey, that really wouldn't be a bad constitutional amendment, at that. Years ago, I used to say that the Seventeenth Amendment was what finally put an end to states' rights." From the ensuing silence, he correctly judged that none of his audience could remember what the Seventeenth Amendment was. "Hey, that's the direct election of senators. Prior to that amendment, United States senators were elected by the state legislatures. You can bet your ass the senate didn't vote any conditional grants in those days. And being a state legislator amounted to more for just that reason. Adlai Stevenson used to say that the state legislatures lost their power because of lack of moral fiber. That's a chump's way of saying he doesn't know what's really going on."

"Okay, you guys," roared O'Toole. "I'll see your ten and raise you ten."

"Call."

"Pass, all around. Let's see your cards."

"I have a flush. All heart, just like myself," said Lien. "Well, O'Toole, what do you have?"

"Full house. Jacks over sevens."

18

Interim Summary

It is now time to make another interim summary of the argument. We have seen that hospitals have many problems which are not directly related to health insurance, but health insurance has invariably applied heat to the pressure cooker. In my opinion, the financing mechanism has created most of the major problems facing hospitals today, and exacerbated most of the rest. The only problem it has mostly solved is the one it was intended to solve— the financial barrier to health care access for most Americans— although we have seen that for some people it actually decreased access. Dealing with the problems of health insurance has thus become one of the embedded problems of American medicine and it has the following ingredients:

- Moral hazard for all four parties in the transaction
- Destruction of the market mechanism for setting prices
- Destruction of power of the consumer to define preferred quality
- Frozen internal organization systems
- Retrospective cost reimbursement
- Excessive inclusion of minor benefit provisions
- Inappropriate secondary enlargement of nonprofit organizations
- Excessive capital expansion and enhancement
- Excessive claims processing cost for small claims
- Proliferation of cost-ineffective technology
- The assignment of benefits

All of these and other points add up to the subtitle of this book, which refers to distortions imposed in the medical system by its financing. The health field has become the second largest industry in the country and a great many people, including physicians, have developed a vested interest in its perpetuation. I have no doubt that this book will make me very unpopular with such people, and I regret it, because they are mostly decent people and it is the system which is at fault, not the people in it. On the other hand, it is my prediction that physicians will be the only group with a vested interest in perpetuating the system who will welcome its reform.

The reason physicians will welcome a sensible reform of the system is that they are beginning to wake up to the fact that they are being drawn into a massive struggle by intruders for control of the second largest industry in the country. Physicians always assumed that they had unassailable credentials consisting of the greatest training in the field, the closest contact with the needs and wishes of the patients, the greatest amount of raw talent as a result of the medical school selection process, and the lifelong habit of working twice as hard as any other occupational group. Having shrugged off the impertinence of other groups for so long, they still find it hard to imagine that bureaucrats, hospital administrators, insurance companies, sociology professors, lawyers, and nurses would have any hope of challenging the primacy of physicians in the physicians' own field. When it is so difficult for physicians to keep up with the knowledge avalanche, how could anyone else hope to do it?

The answer of course is that natural complacency has been augmented by preoccupation with the scramble to stay abreast of the knowledge avalanche, which was also created by insurance money pouring into the system. One of the purposes of this book is to alert physicians along with the public to the fact that moral hazard has been resisted by physicians to a degree that is nowhere matched among competitive components of the system. If we must have moral hazards in the system, the public had better have physicians in charge of it.

In the last few chapters, we examine several solutions which are being proposed, ending with my own. We are sailing under the flag of "all problems are caused by solutions," so it is vital that we pick every nit with innovative proposals for reform lest they, too, become embedded problems. And that includes my own proposals. Certain principles can be laid down:

- Gradual, incremental approaches are much to be preferred to massive reorganizations. We cannot afford to injure a vital commodity like health in disruptive revolutions. We cannot afford to take a chance on monolithic systems which may break down.
- We must not do anything which increases the powerlessness of the patient to define his own best interest himself, or to permit the system to ignore his best interest so defined. The more power that others have, the less power the patient will have. By this I do not mean the general public. Well people are not good judges of how they will feel when they are sick. The repeated history of consumer action groups is that sick people are too busy being sick to get involved, while well people are mainly concerned with keeping their taxes down.
- Imposed non-market constraints on costs invariably affect quality. Not only do the wrong people set priorities in a non-market system but the candy-bar principle applies. The candy bar manufacturer cannot make small increases in prices when the cost of sugar and cocoa rises, because vending machines will only accept dimes and quarters. So the candy bar gets smaller.
- Whenever a proposal is made for reform, we should openly ask who stands to gain from it, and we will usually find that the group who stands to gain will be the one who proposed it. That's not always a thing to be ashamed of. John L. Lewis had a saying that "If a man will not toot his own horn, said horn will not be tooted." But frankness about self-interest will protect us from failing to see that what claims to be a reform is merely a swindle.

In the next chapter we will look at National Health Insurance as exemplified by Canada's experience. The systems in Great Britain and Scandanavia are too alien to have any hope of transportation to this country, but the Canadian experiment is close enough to our system to be politically achievable. The people who stand to gain in such a system are administrators and bureaucrats, as well as the political blocs who imagine that they would have ultimate control.

Following that, we will look at Health Maintenance Organizations (HMO), which carry a great deal of trendiness at present. Since they are little insurance companies, the insurance industry flirts with the idea. Since they generally develop around employer groups, business management perceives the possibility that employers as the fourth-party could control them. Physicians who have been unsuccessful in developing practices see a chance of getting a captive clientele; young physicians are ambivalent about their future prospects, so some of them are attracted.

Next, we look at regulatory approaches, first in the form of patchwork, and then in monolithic regulation. Obviously, bureaucrats and administrators find that to be congenial. Elitists of every background are tempermentally sympathetic with the idea that good should control evil. Thomas De Quincey (in *Confessions of an English Opium-Eater*) had the last word to say about that: "Those of us who enjoy setting things to rights are never much troubled to find that things are wrong."

Finally, the book concludes with my own proposals: To outrage the non-profit hospital system by suggesting that they develop a profit motive, and to restore the market mechanism by tinkering with modifications of high-deductible insurance. My motives are obvious enough. I'm trying to put the patient and the doctor back in charge of their transactions.

19

Groping for Solutions

From an Olympian view, health care has three major components, and there are three massive forces which will shape its future. Health care can be divided into:

1. Routine acute care
2. High-risk ("catastrophe") illness
3. Chronic care

Normally it can be shown that the financial costs of day-to-day routine medical care are bearable for almost everybody, and overinsured for quite a few. It may be true that the rare patient with extraordinary acute costs is not adequately protected against financial catastrophe, and his inability to pay may inflict the financial catastrophe on the institution which tries to help him. It is also definitely true that chronic care is underfunded, and that those who are unfortunate enough to require chronic care are quickly and permanently pauperized. Treated like paupers, too.

In general, if you'd like to know what society wants, you only need to look at what society is doing. Society has apparently decided that members of the productive labor force will be given as much maintenance care as (we hope) is lavished on the airliners we fly. When occasional repair costs vastly exceed the productive value of the individual, we have been inclined to let him take his chances, although as a society we are now considering whether to repair him even when he is totalled. But when it comes to chronic care of lifetime invalids, you had better be either a veteran or a member of a large and wealthy church congregation. The mere fact of your being insane or senile or mentally retarded is not enough for society to act as though it really believed that health care is a right. Sorry about that, but it isn't covered in the program. The British health system made the decision that this inequality wasn't proper, and forcibly diverted funds from acute care to chronic care; but the British public quickly let its rulers know that it wasn't having that. It seems a safe bet that the American public feels the same way.

Now, to turn to the massive forces about to shape our future, some predictions can be made. The population will inevitably become older, and the cost of chronic or custodial care will become a nightmare for society. On the other hand, cheer up; medical science will catch up with the cost of acute care after it passes through the present jumble of new and untried half-successful innovations into another era wherein the treatment of cancer, heart attack, and stroke will be as cheap and simple as treating pneumonia is today. We will, indeed, overcome; research and science are eventually going to solve our acute health cost problems. Our present health financing mess has to be seen as a temporary problem, and not as an interplanetary rocket which will just keep going up forever. Expediency and patchwork, muddling through, may turn out to do the job although possibly not in our generation.

So with the acute care cost problem seen as a temporary phase, it will eventually be replaced by a problem of chronic care cost which is so appallingly large that nobody is presently willing even to face it.

The third massive force which will shape our medical-financial future is the prosperity, or lack of it, of the whole country. British medicine wasn't helped any by the nationalized health scheme, but the basic reason why British medicine is so sad is that England is now almost as poor as Sicily. Some of the developing countries have tried to ignore the hard facts of their situation and nearly ruined themselves. In Liberia, the construction of large modern (i.e., American-model) hospitals has so depleted the country's resources that no money is left for sensible things like maternal and infant care. Countries like Gambia made some harder decisions. Clean the water supply and eradicate mosquito-borne illness, but no money for hospitals. The main hospital in Addis Ababa looks like a summer cottage in the woods, while the teaching hospital in Budapest looks like Bellevue Hospital in 1910. If you want to speculate about who is going to have the best medical care in the world fifty years from now, my guess would be Saudi Arabia. Money talks, and the solutions which America will adopt for its future health-care cost-tangle will bear a heavy relationship to whether our economy expands and booms, or whether we let the Japanese run the world while we relax and admire our traditions.

Canadian Medicine: A Fly Caught in the Amber

One of the few legitimate things to be said in favor of national health insurance is that it amounts to the government deciding to self-insure. In the chapter entitled "Moral Hazards of Third and Fourth Parties," we saw that self-insurance by employers on behalf of their employees' health costs amounted to cutting out the middle man of the third-party. In so doing, the fourth party eliminates marketing costs, the investment of reserves, and insurance company profits. If a contractor is employed to pay claims, competition between contractors may help to control the cost of claims administration. When government not only self-insures but makes self-insurance universal in a country, it eliminates the suspicion that it is subsidizing clients other than its own through the cost-accounting system. However, one has to suspect that even this line of plausible reasoning is erroneous, since the Canadian government has boasted of many features of its scheme but has never claimed that it is cheap to administer. Elimination of subsidies for the uninsured becomes pretty meaningless if everyone is insured, doesn't it?

The Canadian system uses the language and preserves many of the forms of insurance coverage, but all Canadians assume, and no Canadians deny, that health care has become a responsibility of government. Public donation to hospitals dried up immediately after passage of the act and public interest in health exclusively took the political route. In a very short time, political realism on the part of the Canadian public discovered the flaw in the earlier argument that "transfer of medical care from the private to the public sector should not increase its cost." The flaw was that in the public sector, medical care has the appearance of being free, unlimited in extent, guaranteed as to quality. These proved to be costly illusions, and the history of Canadian medicine since the introduction of the health system has primarily been that of government to attempt to constrain the medical budget with the least amount of public outcry. Things have now progressed to the point where it is difficult for a visitor to Canada to find a government official or a member of the health care community who will defend the Canadian system. And yet it is equally difficult to find disagreement with the observation that the illusion of free care is so popular with the public that major reversals of the system are unimaginable without first staging a huge and probably unpopular public education effort.

THE BUREAUCRATIC CONTROL PROCESS

The Canadian medical scheme uses the terminology of insurance but does not really pretend to be anything but a government-run bureaucracy. It is therefore important to understand a few of the standard processes of bureaucracy. Such as:

1. Bureaucracy never initiates new programs, and believes it has a mandate to prevent programs under its control from developing mini-innovations. Bureaucracies live by the rule that only the political process may innovate. That is, only the legislature and the elected upper layer of the executive branch may "set policy," which is the bureaucratic term for creating new programs or abandoning old ones. This protocol is particularly unsuitable for a scientific professional system.

2. The typical funding cycle of new government programs is one of overgenerous budget at first, later squeezed down to the point where the emaciated program must reappeal for political support. If its political constituency rallies behind it, funds are restored; if its political constituency fails to make itself known, the program dies. Politicians and bureaucrats in Canada were puzzled to find that the medical profession considered this "normal" funding cycle to be a treacherous betrayal of trust, since it is not feasible to turn medical care off and on.

3. Because money trickles from the top down, while information necessary to evaluate the national program can only be meaningfully aggregated at the top, the administrators of a bureaucratic program are the first to prosper and the last to starve. Physicians who have served in the armed forces will recognize the phenomenon. The movie *M.A.S.H.* partly describes how they react to it.

PECULIARITIES OF THE CANADIAN SOCIAL ENVIRONMENT

Americans searching for parallels in the Canadian system should remember that Canada was once invited to join the thirteen colonies in revolt against England, and declined. After the American War for Independence, the rather large Tory population of America emigrated to Canada. In 1960 Canadians knew that England had adopted a national health service, and the example was regarded as favorable. England had a frankly socialist government. Socialized medicine was not necessarily a bad thing to Canadians, so national health insurance was not automatically condemned for the possibility that it might lead to socialized medicine.

In the middle west of Canada, roughly to the north of Minnesota, the large Scandinavian population had developed a flourishing farmers cooperative movement with some degree of sympathy to collectivist views of the Scandinavian variety.

And in the Maritime, far northern and far western portions of the country, a small population was stretched over vast expanses of territory. The tradition of generous sharing of resources for common survival was well developed. All of these cultural traditions made Canada more sympathetic to Fabianism, the Webbs, and the London School of Economics than America had ever been. Add to that a strong Canadian sense of fair play: Our government would never trick us.

HOW IT WAS DONE

One must reluctantly confess admiration for the political virtuosity demonstrated by the enactment of the Canadian health scheme. An accommodation was made with every potential source of opposition, each of which found it expedient to accept what was offered. In return for withdrawing from the health insurance market, the commercial insurance companies were allowed to keep their accumulated reserves. The nonprofit Blue plans were promised that they would be used to process claims for the national health scheme (the arrangement lasted only two years, however), while their reserves were turned over to the hospital association as a kind of endowment fund. The medical schools and teaching hospitals received budgeted teaching grants so that they no longer needed to work such costs into the patient care budget (and the patient care cost was thus made to seem smaller). Local politicians had the burden of welfare medical costs lifted from their budgets; they also were given a crucial role in hospital construction control, with 75 percent federal matching money. The medical societies were given a significant power role in a quasi-regulatory body called the College of Physicians and Surgeons. The practicing physicians received a 25 percent increase in fees. Elaborate grievance and negotiating systems were established (described in retrospect as the "process by which creeping socialism creeps"). The public received a promise of unlimited medical care without a financial barrier (but which since has developed many limits, and an increasing number of nonfinancial barriers.)

Such were the details of the interest group bargaining. The political vehicle was the passage of a law which was to remain inactive until a majority of provinces created health schemes. When the majority was reached, those provinces with medical schemes would begin to receive 50 percent matching federal funds. Beginning with Saskatchewan, the proponents of the system concentrated on persuading one provincial legislature at a time to go along. When the time came that only one province more was needed, pressure was applied to Ontario with particular intensity, eventually coming down to a handful of wavering individual politicians. As soon as Ontario entered the system, federal funds began to flow to the provinces which had signed up. Since the holdout provinces were then paying federal taxes to support the schemes of other provinces without receiving federal benefits themselves, they quickly fell in line. The system was nationwide.

LESSONS TO BE LEARNED

1. *The issue is political.* Not economic, scientific, humanitarian, or professional. It is very difficult to find a knowledgable Canadian who will hesitate to identify still more criticisms. The naive American question of why the system persists in spite of its flaws is met with Canadian disbelief, and it is quite clear that no effective means has been found to convince the Canadian voting public that they made a serious mistake.

Bankers talk to other bankers about the inflationary consequences, administrators trade jokes about fiscal crunches, the doctors have found themselves unable to innovate and progress professionally. But so far, the politicians have been successful in picturing the critics as self-seekers, and the criticisms as incomprehensible. There isn't much there that is newsworthy. So the message that the Canadian health scheme is relentlessly inflationary and degrades the quality of care is met with a cynical answer: Maybe so, but the voters like it.

2. *National systems are inflationary.* The insurance mechanism always seems to raise the cost of whatever it touches. But this is not quite the whole story, since if A costs more, you have less to spend on B, so the price of B has to come down. True inflation results from the creation of more money, causing the price of everything to rise. The Canadian experience illustrates, but few Canadians understand, that local or provincial health insurance was not truly inflationary. When the same scheme is federalized it becomes gasoline poured on the general inflationary flames, since only the federal government can print money. So, the liberal Canadian reformers were able to point to the reasonably benign inflation of the provincial health schemes, and were probably honestly unprepared for the inflationary surge which followed the enactment of federal fund-matching.

3. *The quality of care gets worse but it's hard to prove.* The first, last, and perhaps only lesson from Canada is that the politicians come to feel that political popularity is the only useful test of health issues. Every politician faces a rival in the next election; the rival will be delighted to try to demonstrate that a policy was dead wrong. The failure of such demonstration to unseat the proponents of the Canadian health scheme could be taken to mean that the policy can be safely endorsed. But a fair test has not been made, since the Canadian health community has been talking to itself instead of to the public, and has been politically inept in identifying evidence which supports its views.

When concessions were exacted at the start of the system, the concessions should have led to the establishment of an impartial monitoring system to analyze how the experiment was going (instead of merely the concession of an evanescent fee increase). With such an information system it would have been possible to quantify the claims that health administration became bloated, innovation ceased, research declined, teaching was neglected,

Canadians were deprived of many health services available south of the border, and other assertions which now have the sound of unverifiable grousing. If these things are true they will eventually become visible by exploding, but that can't happen in time to discipline the politicians who set it all in motion. Meanwhile the problems will worsen.

4. *Research and innovation are the first to suffer.* Since Canada has now experienced a severe inflation in medical costs (both caused by and causing inflation of the economy), the rationing clamps have been applied hardest on the elements of the health system where there is least immediate impact on voters, and where even the long-run harm is difficult to identify. Research scientists are so far the only professionals in the medical community who have been driven to emigrate in appreciable numbers. New programs of proven value, like diagnostic ultrasound, have not been permitted even in some medical school teaching centers. Most American physicians would recognize the inappropriateness of this policy, and most American voters would not know what was being talked about. If there were no parallel American system for contrast, it would be difficult even for physicians to be sure the policy was having practical adverse effects.

5. *Fixed average fees produce distortion in availability of care.* Since regulatory constraints are the inevitable consequence of destroying the market mechanism, Canada has a fee schedule for physician services. As the physicians came to feel that fees were unjustly low, they responded by increasing the number of simple services and by avoiding the difficult, time consuming ones. (Note the candy-bar principle.) Behaving as any rational person would do in the same circumstances, they sought out situations in which they were likely to perform many repetitive simple tasks, since the fee was the same as for a difficult problem. There is of course an ironic justice that the hypochondriac who had been enthusiastic for unlimited free medical attention quickly found himself unable to obtain any attention or civility at all. But there is a darker side to the perversion of incentives to the point that the physician truly finds it to be against his interest to spend more time on more serious problems. Among the undesirable consequences is a promotion of specialization and subspecialization, since it sometimes becomes possible to claim greater complexity of case load

because of greater complexity of the physician's training. There is certainly no doubt that a fixed fee, particularly an inadequate one, creates an incentive to refer difficult cases to someone else.

6. *Rationing of senior resident physicians adds to inefficiency.* Most lay people would not be expected to comprehend the vital role performed by the senior hospital resident, particularly in surgical and surgical specialty departments. Severe limitation in the number of such positions constricts the production of specialists, which may have been the original intent. However, it also strikes at the heart of the modern hospital care system. There seems to be growing agreement that limitation of senior residents is the mechanism whereby the British medical system can keep 600,000 patients on the waiting list while running 80 percent occupancy. It also bolsters those who claim the doctors are lazy.

The senior residents are, in fact, generally refusing to compromise their standards of quality. The obvious way to break the bottleneck is to allow the work to be performed by junior residents. Or interns. Or nurse practitioners.

7. *After flourishing briefly, medical teaching declines.* Teaching is like research in that it takes a long time for a deterioration to become obvious to the voting public, and is so difficult a subject to quantify that the damages may never be blamed on the politician or bureaucrat who caused them. Ever since the time of Sir William Osler, medical educators have prized the role of full-time (i.e., nonpracticing) teacher. The Canadian scheme provided extra funds for medical teaching, and many new full-time positions were created. However, in time the practicing part-time teachers found that all of their energies were needed just to make a living. The part-timers tended to take their patients with them to the suburbs, leaving the medical school hospitals embarrassed with vacant beds. The full-time physicians increasingly had to work in practice groups, had fewer residents to share either teaching or practice chores, and saw their research funds dry up. Meanwhile, the medical students had decreasing contact with role model doctors who had ever really practiced medicine.

8. *The primary care physician is king.* While it is true that primary care remuneration has been favored in Canada in order to correct a shortage of primary care physicians, there is a political reality to consider. Most primary care physicians have permanent,

long-term relations with several thousand patients. Furthermore, most of their patients are still well enough to go to the polls to vote. Such patients may be locally influential newspaper editors, or ministers, or even politicians. In the small town, there may be no other doctor.

One suspects that these factors play a role in the fact that the primary care physician is the best treated of any provider in the Canadian health scheme. Best treated and least dissatisfied. He is being urged by his specialist colleagues to "opt out" of the system, so far without much effect. His decisions and behavior in the next few years surely are the key to where Canadian medicine is headed.

9. *The doctor must be paid by the patient.* After a bitter strike, during which planeloads of English physician strikebreakers were flown in, Canadian physicians achieved the right to practice outside the health system, sending bills for whatever the patients would agree to pay. The patients were in turn permitted to collect the fixed-fee schedule from the government. As it happens, only 12 percent of Canadian physicians have exercised this right to "opt out" of the system, and most of those who did so were big-city specialists. Specialist physicians have the least political clout, and the greatest dependence on hospitals, and the largest fees, so they must feel fairly desperate to take the chance of refusing the assignment of claim benefits. It is probable that they will be the next group to emigrate if they fail to obtain some relief; if that should happen, it may be possible to quantify the resulting decline in quality of Canadian medical care.

What seems to be happening here is that the family physicians have responded to that incentive to refer difficult cases to specialists which is created by an inadequate fixed-fee schedule. The specialists in turn find they can not make a living on low fees for such selectively difficult cases. Unfortunately, comparatively few Canadian physicians seem to recognize that refusing assigned payments is the proper stance toward the moral hazard of universal insurance. There are now vast numbers of Canadian physicians who have never sent out a bill, and large numbers of Canadian citizens who feel that doctors should not charge for their services. We see the same process at work in American ghetto areas under the Medicaid system.

American physicians, unthinkingly accepting assignments from Blue Shield and Medicare, need to think things through themselves. There seems to be some inclination in Congress to remove the option for American physicians to accept or reject assignment. Disregarding or being unaware of the experiences of claims supervisors that assignment has only marginal administrative advantages for the carrier, Congress may pass such a law. There has to be concern that one of the most abrasive features of the Canadian system could be exported without searching examination.

10. *Facts are obscured by simplified accounting.* Hospitals in Canada are paid on a lump sum basis. It seems to Canadian officials that it would be a useless exercise to prepare itemized bills that are not paid; equally useless, they feel, would be the elaborate process of American-style cost-accounting. Unfortunately, the Canadians (like the British and the U.S. Veterans Administration) have found that an organized health system results in just as much escalation of costs as an unorganized one, with the additional disadvantage of a loss of quality and amenity. Since there was no financial incentive to analyze costs in detail, the Canadians now have difficulty telling a visitor just why their system costs so much. And the doctors have a great deal of trouble accepting the word of their hospital administrators that valid medical programs are being put ahead of valid administrative ones. When you see two hospitals, both of which have indoor swimming pools, neither of which has diagnostic ultrasound equipment, you itch to look over their books. Even without a useful cost accounting, it seems a fair surmise that Canadian medical priorities are not being set by physicians.

HMO: Risk Taking by Physicians?

The great recent concern about rising health care costs among fourth-party employers and government has led to the convocation of an enormous number of public discussion panels on the subject. Such panels typically include a labor leader, a businessman, an economist, and a hospital representative. No matter what constituency or political coloration is represented, such panels typically take only about twenty minutes to agree that the moral hazard of widespread health insurance is the major cause of the recent escalation of medical costs. Naturally it follows that the solution must be some modification of the insurance mechanism, but almost no one on a public panel is willing to see health insurance abandoned. For a while, prepaid salaried group practice arrangements like Kaiser-Permanente were proposed, but government quickly lost interest when it became clear that such groups could anticipate a front-end startup cost of at least $5 million each; subsidizing the seed money for a thousand of those didn't sound like a good way to save money.

Attention then began to turn to certain prepaid insurance arrangements created in central California by groups of physicians who wished to compete with Kaiser, but who also wanted to preserve independent fee-for-service practice. In small towns, the entire medical society might join the arrangement and practice as before, with two changes. The doctor would bill the insurance carrier instead of the patient, and the patient (or his employer) would pay an annual lump-sum premium. On examination, it was found that such arrangements did result in a reduction of hospitalization rates for the subscribers; the doctors and the patients seemed happy, and start-up costs were small. Because clients of the prepaid arrangements were intermingled with the other fee-for-service patients in the doctor's practice, the scheme could start small and grow as fast or slowly as it pleased. If the fee-for-service clients began to find that the pre-paid premium was cheaper, they might switch to it. If the reverse was true, the thing would die and no great harm would be done. Maybe this was a way to change the rules in the middle of the game. If several competitive pre-paid schemes started up in the same locality with different alliances of doctors, maybe this was a way of re-introducing competition into the health field. Competition over the price of the pre-paid premium rather than the price of the service was the goal, and it was linked to the concept of the physician group responding to risk. More money for them if they were careful of patient expenses, less money if they got careless.

All this sounded like a feasible proposal, so the concept of the Health Maintenance Organization (HMO) was born, and federal grants became available to assist with planning and start-up. The California concept was modified somewhat. An HMO was to be a nonprofit insurance company with a mandated majority of nonphysicians on the board of directors, but it would negotiate with an Independent Practice Association (IPA) which could well consist totally of physicians. Each had the freedom to become dissatisfied with the other and seek alternative relationships. In 1979 there were eight million subscribers to prepaid groups (four million of them in California, however), and there is considerable interest among both physicians and employers in learning more about HMOs. Unfortunately, the appraisal on balance is negative.

Inducing doctors to join. HMOs justify their claim of "health maintenance" because failure to maintain subscriber health would theoretically be expensive for doctors instead of lucrative for them. A model might be the mythological Chinese system of paying the doctor only when the emperor was well, and beheading the doctor when the emperor died.

It can plausibly be argued that the Chinese system shortened the life expectancy of physicians without appreciably increasing the longevity of emperors. Surely the Chinese system increased the cost of medical care, and caused a loss of medical quality, since no doctor who was sensible would agree to such a system of risks and rewards. We thus come to the first problem of HMOs: The potential risks are greater than the potential rewards for those physicians whose practice income is already adequate. An under-writing loss of 30 percent might wipe out a year's net income, but a gain of 30 percent more gross revenue means more taxes (certainly) and overhead (probably). The public is thus often put in the position of switching to nonestablished physicians, since HMO marginal economics work in favor of a nonestablished doctor, but work against established ones.

Distorted Patient Mixtures. Indeed, the awkwardness develops that an HMO could not afford to accept an established busy physician anyway, because he would bring along his patients. Such sorted-out subscribers would be considerably more unhealthy, hence more expensive, than the healthy bulk of the population who are not currently seeing a doctor. If an HMO is going to work for Chinese emperors, it would prefer to select healthy ones.

The incentives for the fourth party paying the premium go quite the other way. An employer, of course, has whatever employees he has, sick or well. The premium is mostly experienced-adjusted in his present employee group health insurance, anyway. However, the HMO system does nothing to mitigate the present employer incentive to refuse employment to sickly people, and it may well consolidate the data about his employees' health in such a way as to intensify this antisocial incentive.

Medicare and Medicaid have a worse problem. They have tried to help the HMO program along by exploring the idea of offering to pay an HMO, which accepts their clients, a fee equal to 95 percent of Medicare's average client cost. Superficially, that would sound like a 5 percent bargain until you consider that the HMO has an incentive to select out only healthy clients. Such a process would eventually raise the total government cost quite a bit, since inexpensive well people would likely develop costs below average, while the patients with above-average costs who remained behind in the present system would continue to be just as expensive as ever.

It is unnecessary for the HMO to employ any sly techniques for screening out bad risks, because sick people can be expected to stay with their present physician relationships. A disproportionate number of non-sick would be drifting about, ready to become HMO subscribers.

Small is dangerous. Note also that the risks are safely insurable only if the subscriber group is large. Even a large group would take a few years experience to catch up with pre-existing conditions, and the initial flurry of novelty-seeking. If the subscriber group proves to be unusually unhealthy, what then? It will be interesting to see if anyone will try to bring off a maneuver which has been rumored in the investment mutual fund management field. Keep starting new ones, since eventually you will have a success. (The successful one can boast of its track record, while the unsuccessful ones are dissolved.)

A further problem occurring when an HMO is new and small is that it cannot compete with established businesses for a limited pool of talented managers. The economies of scale are of course missing in small new enterprises, too, so they have to economize on management salaries. A non-profit corporation cannot offer incentive stock options, and in any event nonprofit corporations are perceived by prospective executives as apt to encounter future regulation of management perquisites even when they grow to be big and successful.

Basic Problems of Success. The list of reasons why HMOs have trouble getting started could be expanded further. However, young struggling organizations often create problems for themselves and society by preoccupying themselves so much with the possibility of failure that they fail to forsee what they may encounter should they be so lucky as to succeed in what they are trying to do. There are enough of the original founders of Blue plans still alive, for example, to verify that never did they conceive of the possibility that one day they might become monopolies. Since the HMOs cannot be expected to have any greater foresight, society must consider future issues on their behalf. The significant concerns are:

1. *How are the premiums set?* New, struggling HMOs know that premiums have to be set by guessing. The average costs of Medicare and Medicaid are known, and if you think you can live with 95 percent of that, you take a chance on it. An employer's experience-rated group is easier; you try to come as close to prevailing rates as the employer will allow, and you gamble that you can reduce hospitalization enough to compensate for the initial flurry of novelty-seekers. For the general public, the Blue plan non-group rates are known. You give it a shot, and if federal subsidies won't cover any short-falls, you go bankrupt.

On the other hand, if the HMO survives its initial birth struggles, it can expect inflation to push up its costs, the transient nature of American life to shift the patient mixture, and aging of the population to worsen risk experience. At first, there may be some water in the system which utilization committees can squeeze out, but eventually the hospital prices begin to rise. There is the danger that while the IPA can cut the number of hospital blood counts in half, there is nothing to prevent the hospital from doubling the price of blood counts. A retrospective cost-reimbursement system would in fact tend to force that to happen.

So the HMO eventually has to apply to the insurance commissioner for a premium increase. Experienced insurance companies can attest that there is absolutely no guarantee that a politically motivated insurance commissioner will grant permission for a premium increase, no matter what statistics are displayed for him. So now you have a problem. Why did this organization have to organize as an insurance company? To get federal subsidies, that's why. But in retrospect, it might seem far better to have incorporated the IPA as a medical practice corporation. That way it could charge an annual retainer, as many law firms are accustomed to doing.

Furthermore, either an HMO or a retainer-charging practice corporation might someday grow to the point of monopoly in its area. What regulation would result is unpredictable but it is easy to see that many communities which can justify only one hospital could probably also only justify one HMO. In large metropolitan settings, the pattern of one hospital for one HMO might emerge. In that case, the premiums for each HMO would parallel the premiums for each hospital. The teaching hospital would then be in great jeopardy, and if the insurance commissioner held down fees, the jeopardy would be extreme. Suppose we solved the financial problem. Do we really want to create a system in which rich people go to one hospital and poor people go to another?

2. *How are fees set?* In its inception, the HMO must promise doctors their present fee structure, or doctors won't join. In time, we can expect disputes between doctors about fairness in splitting up the pot. So long as HMOs are small fish swimming in a fee-for-service ocean, the surgeons will tell the pediatricians that they must agree to prevailing surgical fees or do without surgeons. Since the clients would desert if they were unable to get all of their promised services, the threat would be sufficient.

But look ahead to the possibility that the whole community might get absorbed in one or more prepayment schemes. The marketplace would then disappear, and there would no longer be a prevailing fee structure to which disputing specialists could refer. Of course, that would secretly please the lower-paid physicians enormously, especially if they were numerous and fees were voted on.

But it would not ultimately be a good thing for society. I am not a surgeon, and there are times when I resent the higher fees my surgical colleagues and classmates can command. Indeed, to the extent that surgical fees are higher than internist's fees because theirs are covered by insurance and mine are not, I would agree that they are too high. But in saner moments, I must remember that surgical fees were high even in the old days when all patients paid cash. The public acknowledged in a very tangible way that added responsibilities, skill, and reputation were worth something.

Take away that factor, and in time the nation will be asking why it has a surgeon shortage.

An equally serious problem in equity will come in dealing with that great subcontractor of HMOs, the hospital. Are hospitals to bill the HMO their charges, or their retrospective costs?[1] If charges, will those charges be cost-related, or fanciful? If the HMO is to pay costs, how much control will it have over the creation and assessment of indirect costs? If there are coinsurance charges, will the hospital make an effort to collect them, or does it hold the HMO responsible for bad debts? Is the HMO expected to pay for bad debts of its subscribers on personal items? Since the HMO probably will have youngish subscribers, will the hospitals accord the HMO a nursing care cost differential of, say, 91.5 percent? Will there be a charge to the HMO for nonreplacement of blood provided by the Red Cross? How is capital depreciation to be charged? What happens to early-life cash flow surpluses? Will HMOs be forced to consider the ownership of a captive hospital? In short, if doctors are to be at financial risk, they had better define all of the risks they are facing.

3. *How do you keep the candy bar from getting smaller?* Let's be frank about this. American society has gone through a period during which it saw the advances of medical science as a miraculous benefit, in a context of the richest nation on earth becoming even richer indefinitely. We are now recognizing that our exuberance has been a little juvenile, and we are starting to revert to our earlier tradition of the sly Yankee trader. Indeed, it is prudent that we reconsider our attitudes, before the sly Japanese, German, and Arab traders take our hide off. Excellent medical care of our production workers decreases our export prices, but excellent medical care of everyone else is a consumer luxury. We will straddle the issue as long as we can, but if the economic situation really gets ugly, we might have to ration medical care.

To continue to be frank, it is perfectly obvious to our political leaders that a widespread or even universal HMO system would be a workable way to ration care, carrying the political advantage that the doctors would take the blame for the resulting inequities which are also obvious to politicians. The code word for delivering substandard care as a rationing device is "under-utilization." The

1. See Chapter 6, "The Muddle of Hidden Subsidies."

HMO is an excellent way to promote it, since by raising or lowering the permissible prepaid premium, medical care might be turned off and on as the economic climate dictates. The fact that employee groups would aggregate in HMO's might even create a mechanism for maintaining the health of production workers, while rationing medical care for everyone else.

If you prefer some other consumer luxury to be rationed first, you had better hope that utilization committees will be more successful than they have been so far in finding ways of detecting and preventing under-utilization. The utilization review movement has operated on the assumption that society demands curtailment of under-utilization, and so far that has been correct. But every impoverished nation in the world is quite brutal about enforcing selective under-utilization, and it is not safe to assume that America would be different. We should hesitate a moment before we make it too easy to do.

Before HMOs can be permitted to approach a monopoly on medical care, effective ways must be found to show the public what impact its financial policies are having on the quality of that care. If we must reduce the size of candy bars, let's be sure that everybody knows it, and that the decisions are subjected to open adversary process.

SUMMARY AND OVERVIEW

The HMO concept solves two problems: how to make fee-for-service practice (for those who prefer it) competitive with closed-panel salaried[2] practice, and how to restrain somewhat the moral hazard of health insurance. These are considerable achievements, but the HMO concept is flawed by its inability to define a fair insurance premium, its inability to control the prices of hospital services (since the hospitals will curtail teaching and innovation if it tries), and its failure so far to devise an acceptable means of preventing under-utilization. If an HMO system is rapidly established by government subsidy and regulation, those three basic flaws will surface explosively. On the other hand, if the process of HMO establishment is gradual (and tolerated by the medical profession because some alternative seems worse), then the three

2. The Kaiser System pays doctors salaries, and selects a limited (closed) panel of them for the patient to choose from. Kaiser is the salaried closed panel prototype.

central risks will present themselves as imbedded structural problems for future generations to view with frustration. Complex systems take a long time to change.

Perhaps it would be well to ask ourselves just what we hope to achieve with an HMO. The present federal emphasis is on inflation control, and thus on cost containment. Since the only provable benefits of HMOs lie in reducing the use of in-patient hospital care, perhaps it would be best to see HMOs as only one of several ways to reduce in-patient hospital usage. There are other ways.

The subscribers to Philadelphia Blue Cross have experienced a 30 percent reduction in hospital days (from 1,085 days per thousand subscribers to 760 per thousand) in eight years. Since the West Coast group practices can only claim to have reduced hospitalization to 550 days per thousand in twenty years, perhaps things are not so desperate as they seem. The PSRO in Philadelphia has apparently achieved a reduction of 4 percent in the last year. Instead of focusing on the distraction that 4 percent reduction in hospitalization only causes a 1.5 percent reduction of true costs, perhaps we should notice that 4 percent per year will get us down to the HMO level in another eight years. Without disrupting the present structure of medical care, and without locking us into a monolithic payment system which would create some novel unpleasant surprises of its own.

Six Other Misguided Proposals

Let's get back on the track. HMOs are going nowhere at the moment, and the prevailing mood in Congress is that national health insurance would bankrupt the country. We will soon examine the regulatory approach to restraining health costs, which appeals to those who hope that vigilance and selective coercion by an elite would restrain the weaknesses of the multitude. If our problem is high costs, let's hold costs down. Before we examine massive regulation, however, let us first look at patchwork regulation. Our problem, remember, is to cope with the inherent problems of our present system of health insurance.

Five currently popular suggestions for reform of the system, and one covert one, have been tried and found wanting. They fail because they only address superficial manifestations of hospitals rather than underlying reimbursement issues.

1. *Eliminate trivial or unprofessional hospital admissions.*
There is no doubt that reduction of hospital admissions would
slowly reduce health costs. By that is meant alternative delivery of
care in less expensive settings. However, Professional Standards
Review Organizations (see the next chapter) have progressed
sufficiently in their survey of current medical practice habits to
encourage confidence that the vast bulk of current hospital admissions are for legitimate purposes in the existing environment of
alternatives.

Some questionable admissions have of course been uncovered.
Such cases as have been found were usually quite brief admissions,
implying that mistakes were quickly rectified. Almost by definition, unnecessary admissions have less "intensity of service." That
is, each day of care is simpler and cheaper than is true of necessary
admissions. Hence, their elimination would result in a longer
average length of stay, and a higher average daily room charge, for
patients in general. If you could eliminate unnecessary admissions
completely without even greater cost in monitor effort, the savings
to the community would be reflected in a reduction of the number
of "in-patient claims" per year, per thousand population, but the
dollar savings might not be proportionate. Truly appreciable reduction of hospital admissions would require some expenditure for
the provision of treatment alternatives, and a certain hidden cost of
re-educating patients and doctors to new practice patterns. Shifting
the locus of care will slowly pay big dividends. Chasing the rascals
out is an illusion.

2. *Reduce the length of hospital stay.* PSRO review has
definitely shown, however, that a very considerable number of
patients who need to be admitted to the hospital do stay there
longer than they really need an acute care facility. This, too, is a
more complicated issue than it sounds. A few people do abuse their
insurance by insisting on staying until their relatives can pick them
up on Saturday, and some doctors are overcautious in discharging
people who could perfectly well go home. But many other delays
are caused by internal scheduling tangles which would require
quite a disruptive reorganization to ameliorate. Finally, there are
the people, particularly in large urban hospitals, for whom no
acceptable cheaper alternative exists in the community.

There has been a very large flight of medical care to the suburbs.

Along the beltway around Washington, D.C., for example, new hospitals are sprouting like mushrooms. Naturally, this migration has left surplus hospital capacity behind in the center of the city. Never mind for a moment that this inflexibility is attributable to the non-profit nature of center-city hospitals. The present point is that there really is no sense in building nursing homes in the urban centers when the same function could be performed in the surplus acute care beds. Our exasperating cost-reimbursement system makes it appear as though subacute patients are costing society $200 or more every day they stay in the acute hospital, but that is nonsense. The true cost of the really acute patients is made to look smaller than it really is, by the enforced averaging of costs for everyone in a bed. When cost containment measures are proposed, urban hospitals become terrified that they will be trapped within artificially low average costs, and then somehow be deprived of the low-cost subacute patients who depressed the average.

Of course the silly reimbursement system needs to be changed; that's what this book has said a hundred times. But here we need to make the negative point that shortening the average length of stay by discharging half-well people is monstrous. Closing surplus hospital beds at the same time you build new nursing homes is madness.

Meanwhile, the painful slow process of streamlining the flow of activity during the process of cure is gradually shortening the average length of stay at a rate of about 4 percent per year. But statistics strongly suggest that reducing the volume of care isn't solving the cost problem. Look at the 1978 annual report of Philadelphia Blue Cross:

YEAR	AVERAGE DAILY HOSPITAL CHARGES GREATER PHILADELPHIA AREA
January 1977	$225
January 1978	258
January 1979	300

Dividing the claims incurred by the number of subscribers, we see what it cost in premiums to have 30 percent less hospital care:

YEAR	DOLLAR COST OF CLAIMS INCURRED PER SUBSCRIBER
1974	$100
1975	120
1976	138
1977	155
1978	170

Now it is true that there was a considerable extension of Blue Cross out-patient benefits during the time in question. However, the argument for extending those benefits was that it kept people out of the hospital, and hence saved money. Did it?

3. *Reducing the volume of services.* The reader has now been dragged to the idea that the cost of hospital care has been shooting up while at the same time the doctors have effected a marked decrease in hospital bed usage. The insurance companies who are in a position to observe the externals of this process call it an increase in the "intensity" of hospitalization. From this phrase, it is an easy logical leap to assume that new high technology (i.e., CAT Scanners) and overuse of old small technology (i.e., duplicate laboratory examinations) account for the cost rise. Not so.

The escalation of hospital cost has occurred disproportionately in the indirect component of costs, rather than in direct costs such as new technology, new drugs, and laboratory procedures (necessary or unnecessary). Take the matter of drug costs, for example:

MEDICAL CARE COMPONENT OF CONSUMER PRICE INDEX
(1967 = 100)

YEAR	SEMIPRIVATE ROOM	PRESCRIPTION DRUGS
1967	100	100
1968	114	98
1969	129	100
1970	145	101
1971	163	101
1972	174	101
1973	182	101
1974	202	103
1975	236	109
1976	269	115
1977	300	122

The economic principle reversing the effect of "intensity" is called economy of scale. It costs less per service to perform a large number of services than it did to perform a small number, and the incremental cost of doing one more is usually much less than the average cost of doing them all. You reach a point in automated technology where the incremental cost of one extra test may be only the electricity of running the machine for two minutes. If you don't do the last test, your saving is negligible. And if you do a few extra, the cost is next to invisible.

Any course in freshman college economics teaches the foregoing principle of "marginal economics." What gets renewed emphasis here is the perversion of marginal cost incentives by the nonprofit, cost-reimbursed system. A profit-oriented system makes most or all of its profit in the last 10 percent of sales, and profit-oriented systems are therefore extremely responsive to minor changes in volume. Cost-reimbursed nonprofit systems can afford to be quite relaxed about changes in volume. It doesn't cost much more to be wasteful, and you don't save much by being efficient. When the thrust of national goals was to extend care as much as possible, a cost-reimbursed system was a cheap way to do it. Now that national priorities have shifted to cost-saving, the cost-reimbursed system has to change back to some system where money talks.

4. *The seven-day week.* The Cooper Hospital in Camden, New Jersey actually tried out the attractive idea of a seven-day work-week. What they discovered was that their best employees promptly obtained employment in hospitals with more acceptable "working conditions." The point was quickly accepted in hospital circles that a seven-day week was only workable in areas where there was an oversupply of medical labor. Undoubtedly, a level of overtime pay could be found which would induce anyone to work the graveyard shifts, but the cost would be prohibitive.

It must be conceded that there are many profitable businesses which work a five-day week by choice, within highly competitive environments. The questions are: What is the value of the unused weekend capital capacity, compared to the increased labor cost of off-hours work? Expensive though they may be, hospital buildings and equipment are not in a class with large computer installations where a machine cost of $800 an hour justifies all-night operation. Hospitals are becoming more capital-intensive, but labor costs are still 50 percent of the budget. To look into the future, most of the new employee positions which have been created in the past twenty years in such abundance involve work in forty-hour-week departments. Nursing and medical professions do not relish but do acknowledge a round-the-clock professional obligation. The new-comers to hospital work—in the accounting, laboratory, and ad-ministrative areas—look at things differently, as most Americans do.

One cannot be certain that the nonprofit hospital makes its decisions quite so abstractly, since employee satisfaction counts for a great deal and profit counts for little. For several years, I toured several hospitals on Christmas day, counting empty beds. For the most part, sixty nursing units were half-empty. One suspects that it is not pure economics which prevents the tempo-rary consolidation of vacancies into thirty completely empty units, with furloughed staff.

One further consequence of the annual Christmas emptying of hospitals is a predictable crisis congestion of the same units in January. Most hospitals do not work off this rebound backlog until early March. Dr. Lonnie Bristow of San Pablo, California, has made the ingenious suggestion that hospitals should impose a 20 percent coinsurance surcharge for admission between January 2 and February 15 each year, in order to encourage the shifting of elective patients to other times. Judging from past experience, there would have to be some way to prevent such surcharges from being written off and collected as bad debts. Better than a punitive surcharge system for January would be a reduced-rate incentive for December. But how do you reduce prices for patients who already are fully covered by insurance? Why would they want to spoil their holidays?

5. *Close hospital beds.* By this point, the reader may understand the sense of frustration which overtakes many serious students of hospital cost containment. Nothing works, but something must be done anyway. The more frustrated you get, the more drastic you are willing to become.

So, the idea eventually surfaces that it might be a good idea to create a shortage of hospital facilities. Then let *them* figure out how to get along with less.

Such a bloody-minded attitude is unquestionably now part of the reasoning of many Health Service Administration boards, and it may even have been the Congressional attitude when P.L. 93-641 was passed. If bed limitation would save money, it might be defensible. But it will cost more money. Never mind the considerations of human suffering and rationing of care. Applying the bottleneck approach to hospital beds will explode the financial bottle. Yes, hospital construction is expensive. No, it isn't the biggest cost. We just finished showing that it isn't cost-effective to run a seven-day week. Does it make sense to force a seven-day week to happen?

Take that post-Christmas congestion as a case in point. Do you suppose the average length of stay, corrected for diagnosis, gets longer or shorter in January? If you find an example where it is shorter, what then happens to the average dollars per day or average dollars per case?[3]

The unfortunate consequence of such close-the-beds reasoning is that the hospitals with least political clout are most apt to get closed. As it turns out, such hospitals generally have the lowest costs. Philadelphia has closed a proprietary hospital and its thousand-bed municipal hospital, both of which had costs considerably below average, and their levels of amenity were considerably below that of the other hospitals. The message has to be pretty clear: Build yourself a new expensive building, or get closed up. It remains to be proven that the cost savings, if any, of bottlenecking hospital beds can justify the present panic of facility enhancement.

6. *Create hidden waiting-lists.* Our own management inefficiencies create many situations where the patient stays longer than he would have to if we engineered things better. If these internal delays should be deliberately exaggerated, eventually the hospital bed capacity will become inadequate, even though it is not overtly reduced. Indeed, enough internal bottlenecks already exist so that it is only necessary to be lethargic in identifying and correcting them in order to create the same situation.

People fall into this approach unconsciously depending on the incentives which guide them. It may be that a subordinate hospital

---

3. It happens that I don't know the answer to these questions, which others are challenged to examine. But it scarcely seems like going out on a limb to generalize that a congested system is an inefficient, expensive system. If Congress thought otherwise when it passed P.L. 93-641, Congress had better authorize some research.

It becomes clear that there is a vital public need for a system to be established for monitoring and analysing the delays which a congested hospital system might be creating. Whatever the shortcomings of the British Health Service, it must be admitted that the British have made an aggregated count of their waiting lists, whereas in America it is impossible to say how many patients are currently on standby, what hospitals or regions are in better or worse state of congestion, what types of patients or specialized facilities are in supply or shortage, and how the situation is changing with time.

The medical profession can most reasonably provide the standards by which hospital admission delays can be judged. As a start, let us divide candidates for hospital admission into three classes:

1. *Emergencies.* Defined as patients whose health will suffer from delayed admission.
2. *Urgent.* Defined as patients who would experience real discomfort from delayed admission.
3. *Elective.* All others, not overlooking the consideration that these patients have lives to lead, preferences to express, baby-sitters to arrange, employment coverage to organize, etc., while they are in the hospital. They want to know when to expect admission, and they have a right to have the guarantee honored.

If these definitions can be accepted, it would be a reasonable standard to expect that only a major community disaster would cause an emergency patient to be turned away; that an urgent patient should not wait more then 48 hours; and that a guaranteed elective patient should have his guarantee kept. It is no secret that these standards would be tough for many hospitals to meet, even with a statistical surplus of beds, and it is fairly predictable that a reduction of beds would increase the waiting lists.

employee doesn't strain himself because no one is pushing him. It may be that a chief executive officer puts a low priority on hiring or promoting hard workers when he has more urgent problems. It may be that an insurance company prefers not to rock the boat with hospitals, client companies, or unions. It may be that a legislator or a regulator promotes a pet scheme which has the secondary consequence of tangling up some obscure but vital step in the orderly flow of patient care.

However, the familiar Murphy's Law says that anything which can go wrong eventually will. Someone is bound to see that a proposal masquerading as the diversion of excess specialists to primary care will really slow down elective surgery through the mechanism of reducing the supply of senior surgical residents. No one can be sure that this motivated any Englishman, but this is the British way of rationing health care.

In May, 1978, there were 591,000 patients waiting for admission to British Hospitals; 40,000 of these patients were classified as "urgent". The delays were nonuniform in different geographical areas, with a removal of gall stones delayed four weeks for a London patient and seven years for a patient in a remote province of Scotland. It is generally true throughout Britain, however, that a cataract extraction will be delayed three years from the time of applications. Tory party spokesmen assert that the waiting list grossly underestimates the unsatisfied medical needs of the British community but the official statistics of the Labor Party ministry were quite lurid enough to convince an American that there can be worse things for a community than to be "over-bedded."

Hospitals, after all, are not collections of uniformly interchangeable beds. The hospital is compartmentalized into special units, such as obstetrics and psychiatry, postoperative recovery rooms, adolescent treatment units, special study day care units, burn centers, and emergency triage holding areas. It is of no use to the patient with a heart attack that, although the coronary care unit is full, there are empty bassinets in the newborn nursery. From this specializaton of dedicated treatment units comes the paradox that a hospital can simultaneously have empty beds and a shortage of beds, or that the community as a whole can have chronic bed vacancies while it also has insufficient facilities. In Great Britain there were 383,000 available beds in 1976, with an average occupancy of 311,000 patients, and a waiting list which averaged 607,000 patients in spite of only 81 percent occupancy. In the HEW Secretary's terms, the English provision of 8.4 beds per thousand was more than twice his standard; it would be an interesting experiment to see how long the waiting list would become if England reduced its hospital beds to the HSA guideline of four per thousand population.

Next we will examine more massive regulatory approaches, organized into official bodies or pursuing an official doctrine. The major trouble with having such proposals even on the horizon is that they create an incentive to slow down voluntary self-regulation. They make it seem attractive to put on a little fat for the coming winter.

20

Over Breakfast Coffee

"How far along are you with the book, dear?"

"Most of the way, except for the zingers at the end. Norm Makous suggested yesterday that I put in a jab about gas rationing."

"What in the world does that have to do with medicine?"

"Something to the effect that if the government made a mess of gas rationing, think what a mess they would make of rationing medical care."

"You know, dear, this book has done you a lot of good."

"Well, that surely remains to be seen. What do you mean?"

"It taught you how hard it is for somebody to follow what you are saying."

"Yes, it has taught me what Ben Franklin knew a long time ago. If you want to convince people, don't use logic. Tell stories."

"Tell me another."

"Well, I'm playing around with two of them. The first is the chocolate bar story."

"That may be clear to you, dear, but it isn't clear to everyone."

"Sure. The chocolate bar company has trouble raising prices because the vending machines only take dimes and quarters. So, when the price of sugar and cocoa goes up, what do they do?"

"They make the candy bar smaller. And you're saying that holding down the price of medical care causes the quality to deteriorate. Am I right?"

"Yes, indeed. Fisher's First Law. And now for the IBM story."

"Oh dear. Computers again. Isn't it enough that you got our first son interested in that? Do I have to be interested, too?"

"Of course you are interested. Just listen. The computer programmers have a new generation of programming called distributed processing. Before that, they had a programming generation called real time, which depended on the system called linked lists. But the programmers are just kidding themselves. Those programming generations were merely outgrowths of two engineering generations called silicone chips and telecommunications, respectively. But in turn the electrical engineers are just kidding themselves, too. The real generations in computers grow out of the tax laws. The IRS won't let the customer take a full equipment tax write-off and depreciation unless the machine is kept for seven years. So the customer only has money to spend every seven years. The computer company just holds up whatever technology has appeared in the meantime, and releases it as a new generation every seven years."

"Good heavens. I like the candy bar story better."

"Maybe you do, but the two stories illustrate different points. The candy bar illustrates the unwisdom of restraining prices externally, and the computer story illustrates that unexpected distortions grow out of all laws and regulations."

"You know, dear, the book has done something for me, too. It has taught me that I'm really not so stupid when I can't follow what you're saying."

21

Regulation: Better Is Not Always Best

Thank God for Freddie Laker. Sir Frederick Laker, the British entrepreneur who launched a cheap third-class transatlantic air service, with the rather surprising results that:

1. He became a multimillionaire.
2. The established airline giants of the transatlantic air cartel were forced to lower their prices.
3. The glut of empty seats which had characterized transatlantic air travel promptly turned into a shortage of space as new travelers were able to afford to fly.
4. The Carter administration was then tempted into deregulating American domestic airlines, an action followed by a similar burst of popularity for local air travel.
5. A Democratic administration found itself with its first domestic political triumph, which was a dramatic public demonstration of the general foolishness of public utility regulation.

Earnest reasoning or learned essays could never have had as much effect on public attitudes as Freddie Laker's insolent example, because lots of people fly, and lots of people watched the experiment. Lowered prices made airlines rich. Increased competition led to vastly increased service. More people could afford air travel. International air cartels and domestic airline regulation had, it would seem, been damming up all of those public benefits, and it is not clear in retrospect that anyone at all was served well by the regulation. So there is hope for us all that America's forty-year romance with regulation may be ending.

Note first the essence of Freddie Laker's achievement: He offered low quality at low prices. No crashes, please, but inconvenient hours, bad food, inaccessible ticket counters, unlocatable hangers in strange airports. Freddie Laker gave the term "fly-by-night" a new significance. Like the airlines, the medical establishment has become so intimidated by the holy grail of high quality that we have not noticed how quality has been the stated excuse for every new regulation. We wouldn't want poor quality medical care, now, would we?

Unfortunately, we also don't want to be regulated to death, and a mindless subservience to the intonations of excellence is a perfect legal theory for rule makers to embroider and for the judicial system to enforce. To wit:

1. It lies at the heart of the malpractice crisis.

2. Put yourself in the position of an equipment salesman talking to a hospital purchasing agent who knows his institution will be fully reimbursed; you don't talk price, you talk quality.

3. The community has been convinced it has an excess of hospital beds, but all would still agree that we must upgrade the quality of obsolescent facilities, and close the small low-quality (but low-cost) institutions.

4. Licensing is now not enough; the education industry advocates relicensing on a periodic basis.

5. The staffing of hospitals, to improve quality, shows credentialism gone mad. A radiologist cannot select and promote the technician best qualified in his opinion to be chief technician whenever the technician might not have the specified schooling required by a joint commission or state health regulatory act. Some other technician must be promoted, in spite of demonstrated unworthiness, because the credentials are better.

6. The most determined regulators of all are unions, but even they have learned to conceal self-interest behind the screen of improved patient care.

It would be an interesting thing if someone would carry the quality issue to the Supreme Court. Let us suppose that some hospital or community, denied some medical quality item by some regulatory body, put forward the theory that society had created a money-no-object reimbursement system intentionally, and had relentlessly pursued a coherent pattern of medical money-no-object behavior; therefore, who was the regulator who sought to frustrate the clearly expressed will of the Republic? Health care as a right would then be driven as far as it could go. As Mr. Dooley would have remarked, the Supreme Court would read the election returns and its decision, therefore, would be hard to predict.

We now discuss four regulatory systems which have been proposed for the hospital industry, implemented to some degree, and getting mixed reviews.

PSRO: A Good Idea with Delayed Puberty

The Professional Standards Review Organizations, created in 1972 by Senator Wallace Bennett and the Senate Finance Committee, are outgrowths of a fundamentally sound idea. Recognizing the utter impossibility of deciding medical quality issues by consumer groups, juries, bureaucrats, or legislators, Senator Bennett proposed that they be settled by the collective consensus of physicians in a locality. If a patient's doctor felt that some process was proper, and there was agreement from both the patient (that's known as informed consent) and the physician's local colleagues (that's known as peer review), and no disagreement from colleagues from other regions (the process of monitoring and appeal)—if all of these steps of peer review and due process were in order, then you have done the best you can and you just have to live with the outcome. Senator Bennett said he had a clear recollection of sitting in the operating room many times as a young man in response to an old Utah law which mandated that a relative of the patient must always be on hand, in the room, whenever surgery was performed. His subsequent distrust of such lay review of professional performance was very profound. At the same time, his reservations about the limitations of human nature show through in the carefully considered procedures and safeguards of the act. If the doctor is an imperfect agent, he is nevertheless the best imperfect agent we can train. If society has a problem deciding whether certain health care is substandard in quality, it seems reasonable to ask the opinion of other doctors. Furthermore, if society declares that it will pay for any treatment which is medically necessary, it is also reasonable to ask other doctors whether something was indeed medically necessary.

So the 1965 amendments to the Social Security Act declared:

Medicare and Medicaid would pay for medical care which was medically necessary and of acceptable quality. The 1972 amendments declared: What was quality and what was medically necessary would be defined by local groups of doctors organized in local PSROs, subject to appeal.

It would be very hard for a doctor to reject the reasonableness of the Bennett amendment, and almost no challenge has been made by lay groups. But moral hazard affected doctors and patients less than Congress imagined, and affected institutions and bureaucracies more than was ever dreamed. The PSRO[1] now appears to have had six flaws in its design:

Fault 1. Delegation to hospital staffs. The bill contained a section with the central concept that no doctor in a PSRO would be permitted to review activity in any hospital where he was a member of the staff. Senator Bennett was no fool, and he rightly felt that the review process should be removed from whatever conflicts of interest might exist in an institution, both in the way of undue leniency to friends and in vendettas against competitors. At the very last moment before final passage of the act, a strong lobbying effort by hospital groups succeeded in switching the sense of that section completely. Without bothering to revise the original language, it was interposed that the PSRO must accept the review findings of internal hospital committees, a completely reversed concept. One can hear Senator Bennett's skepticism in a second interpolated clause, "but only if, and only to the extent, and only for such time, as the PSRO is satisfied." Experience has demonstrated that the PSRO has no way to be dissatisfied unless someone complains, or unless a spot-check monitoring process turns up irregularities. Subsequent fiscal starvation of the program has pretty well protected hospitals against excess monitoring, and as far as complaints are concerned, well, who's complaining?

Fault 2. Overlooking the culture shock for the bureaucracy. The authors of the PSRO law apparently greatly underestimated a revolutionary concept of government which was implicitly folded into the statute. The PSRO was not to be a top-down regulatory body; it was to be a complex of 200 independent local corporations who would develop local case law which would eventually coalesce

1. My younger son was overheard explaining to other teenagers that PSRO meant "Physician's something 'r other."

into a medical common law, as different jurisdictions wrestled with the same problems and came to independent conclusions.

If the PSRO system had been placed in the judicial branch of government, the judicial branch would have recognized the parallels and would have known what to do with the PSRO. As it was, the bureaucracy of the executive branch appeared baffled by how to implement the law. A typical reaction was that reported of Elliot Richardson who was Secretary of HEW at the time the law was enacted. He is said to have turned to an aide and reportedly said something like, "Please go over to the Hill and see if you can find out what this thing is all about." It should therefore be no surprise, and it certainly is no dark conspiracy, that the bewildered civil servants at HEW who were given the program to run, adopted a number of conventional bureaucratic approaches which were unintended by the law. Instead of a common law coalescing from the grass roots upward, the PSRO became characterized by a bombardment of transmittals from the top down. Pathetic underfunding of the program tended to force things into a conformist mold anyway, because there was not enough money to pay for the originally contemplated diversity of approach. More skillful bureaucrats would have known how to bludgeon the funds out of OMB (Office of Management and Budget) and the House Appropriations Committee.

For their part, the doctors were inexperienced in the ways and wiles of Washington, did not understand what was being asked of them, and had not asked for the program in the first place. It appeared like some bureaucratic regulatory process to them, since the transmittals and regulations looked like the caricature they had in their minds of a bureaucracy. And then, the crowning insult of not being paid to spend a great deal of time on an uncomfortable task was visited upon them. The hourly rate for physician service time was fairly generous. However, strangulation of the budget reduced the funds for remuneration to so few hours that a federally mandated program had to be conducted in the spare time of semi-volunteer doctors. One typical accommodation was to aggregate available money into a half-time salary for one doctor, to whom the program was then abandoned, and who knew that a time would inevitably come when he would be sniped at for dominating the program, hogging the money, or becoming "just another bureaucrat, himself." All this was happening to a program in which the nation was asking all doctors to help out with their best collective judgment.

As a footnote, however, this floundering minuet of the bureaucracy and organized medicine has set in motion some sociological changes which are probably the most important result of the PSRO program. Organized medicine now has learned what government is all about, and it remains to be seen which of the two will be more altered by the encounter.

Fault 3. Not much to criticize. There had been quite a bombardment of innuendo and even lurid newspaper stories about rich doctors, publication of the names of doctors with large incomes from welfare recipients,[2] Medicaid Mills, and so on. It must indeed be admitted that the medical profession was a little nervous about what might crawl out from under the rock when PSRO review was begun. The economists speak of moral hazard, and Imperfect Allegiance of the Agent, which are nice terms for an ugly problem. Maybe it was going to be a sorry mess.

Well, it wasn't. The fact is now clear that the profession had been somewhat slandered, and that the rising cost of health care could not be attributed to physician fraud and abuse even out in the third decimal.

Fault 4. The frustration of cost reimbursement. If the PSRO found itself with a negligible task in controlling substandard or reprehensible medical behavior, perhaps it could do something about costs created by thoughtlessness and inefficiency. It was here that the PSROs got a lesson in retrospective cost reimbursement which showed them how naive Congress had been, both in 1965 and in 1972.

If the PSRO identified a pattern of unnecessarily protracted hospitalization, its first job was supposed to be education, although it was provided no funds to educate. So it scolded, but eventually had to implement threats and deny payment. It is usual in such cases to find that fault is shared by the patient, the doctor, and the system created by the institution. Sometimes fault is shared by an ambulance service failing to take the patient home, or a nursing

2. In a famous episode, Secretary Joseph Califano had to apologize for publishing a list of doctors who were "ripping off" the Medicaid program for big incomes. In over two-thirds of the cases, it turned out that the doctor was legitimately billing on behalf of a large clinic or hospital and not receiving the income himself.

home not having a vacancy, or the state welfare department not providing funds for a place for the patient to go.

But let us assume that in a given case the hospital is clearly and exclusively at fault for an unnecessarily prolonged hospitalization. Payment might be denied for, say, six days of care at two hundred dollars a day. Who pays for such a loss? The handful of patients who pay their own bills or who are covered by commercial insurance do, and this is accomplished by raising posted charges. So the net result of penalizing a hospital for keeping a Medicare patient too long is to raise the cost of care for another patient who has commercial insurance, and to raise the medical component of the consumer price index without changing medical costs. (See Chapter 7, "A Primer from the Trustees.")

Take it another way. Suppose the educational and peer review process is ultimately successful in reducing the average length of stay of Medicare patients by 20 percent. How much money would be saved? It would be an exaggeration to say none would be saved, but perhaps the correct figure is 6 percent. Since up to 70 percent of the hospital costs are indirect, they continue fixed as before and migrate to other patients. Perhaps the point becomes clearer if you imagine a hospital empty for two days because of a bomb threat. The costs would be almost as much as if the hospital were full. Even if you didn't pay some of the employees, there would still be costs of depreciation, interest, heating, and maintenance of the empty building.

All of this is marginal economics which we all should have anticipated. Gradually the realization is circulating among the medical profession that poor utilization practices couldn't have caused, and didn't cause, the notorious health cost increases of the past twenty years. Consequently, working hard to expedite hospitalization is nice, but it can't possibly save much money. Even if you are successful.

Fault 5. Privileged information. There seems to have developed a substantial literature on the theory and practice of regulation. In that literature, it is regarded as a fundamental truth that the regulator cannot function unless he has access to huge amounts of information. If you want to cheat, in other words, hide.

In the case of medical information, the medical profession is thereby touched at an extremely sensitive nerve. Doctors don't like to poke around in personal data, and they don't want others to do it, either. The point of confidential privilege was not exactly invented recently. Every doctor swears to the Hippocratic Oath which states, among other matters: "Whatsoever things of the affairs of men which I shall learn in the course of my profession, I shall hold forever secret."

Does the public really want to change that? Doctors don't.

Fault 6. How much better is best? So, finally we come back to Freddie Laker, who demonstrated that third-class air travel is something the public needed and wanted, possibly even more.than second-class travel, and certainly more than first-class travel. That free champagne on the Concorde is nice, but safe cheap air travel is better. The Constitution doesn't say that health care is a right, but plenty of voters say it is, so how far do you go with quality?

What we seem to have here is a realization, after seven years of PSRO, that the United States Senate didn't quite get the mission defined correctly. It wanted help with the escalating costs of health care, and it decided to take the advice of the doctors. Unfortunately it was imagined that improper, substandard, or inefficient care would be the principal adverse response to the moral hazard of health insurance. That's wrong. The moral hazard expressed itself in a mindless extension of the idea that nothing is too good for our patients. Even the patients don't always want that. Most old patients have become terrified that someone will subject them to unspeakable tortures and indignities in the intensive care unit, just to keep them alive another month. And their doctor may just do that, too, since society is sending him the signal that if he doesn't, he is liable for a malpractice suit. From issues of this gravity down to whether to raise the head of the bed with a motor or a crank, quality always seems to win.

There are grave doubts in this author's mind that anything short of abolishing retrospective cost reimbursement will help restrain cost-free perfectionism, but at least the PSRO might be encouraged to turn its attention to the issue. Surely it is true that society needs the advice of its best-trained profession in deciding where to draw the line. Even if the result is only another demonstration of the futility of regulation, the education of both profession and public would prepare the way for consensus.

HSA: Regulation By the Planning Process

Let us put some facts side by side:

1. In 1968 the American Hospital Association indicated support for comprehensive health planning and developed a model certificate-of-need law. The idea did not originate at that time, but had been discussed within the organization and partly implemented in several states before 1968.

2. In 1974 Congress passed P.L. 93-641, the National Health Planning and Resources Development Act, which mandated the creation of local Health Systems Agencies (HSA) who recommend[3] approval of new capital expenditures for health in their areas.

3. The history of the planning process has demonstrated that HSAs are disinclined to permit new entrants into the hospital marketplace.

4. The history also demonstrates that most applications for enhancement of existing hospitals are approved, and indeed the recent wave of hospital building programs is astonishing. The Chicago HSA has approved 52 of its 55 applications, for example.

5. Most HSA regions are large enough so that there often exist local areas of bed shortage within regions which have a general bed surplus, or areas of surplus next to areas of shortage. Instead of following the market signals which would allow the most crowded hospital to enlarge and an empty one to close, there has been a tendency to give a little to everybody.

6. There has been a strong "tar-baby effect," in which it is proposed to extend "certificate-of-need" legislation to areas which might complement or supplement (or compete with) hospitals, such as nursing homes and doctor's offices.

FAILURES OF THE PLANNING PROCESS

The framers of the HSA law were acutely conscious of the possibility of medical-care-provider domination of the program, so

---

3. The HSA recommends to the State Health Coordinating Council (SHCC), which finally approves. The history of support or rejection of HSA recommendations by the SHCC has been quite nonuniform.

board and committee memberships are limited by law to a trivial number of providers. A nonprovider of health care is sometimes defined as someone who derives less than 10 percent of his family income from the health industry. This puritan concept could be carried to the point of disqualifying a shoemaker whose wife worked part-time as a typist for Blue Cross. Experience under some older planning agencies had amply demonstrated that something like this had to be done, since some of those agencies could have given lessons in logrolling to Lyndon Johnson.

So, after the first few meetings, no one wants to be a member of an HSA Board of Directors except:

1. Providers, who are severely limited
2. Consumer groups, with a clear prejudice in favor of internal subsidies for their pet schemes or ethnic groups
3. Unions, with one eye on subsidies and the other eye on unionizing hospital employees
4. Local governments, looking to improve the local economy with construction and added employment
5. Would-be influence peddlers
6. And just plain egomaniacs

In practice, it is alarming to see that most HSA decisions are heavily influenced by who is making the proposal. It would seem that a community might or might not need a new capital project. Therefore, it is a little puzzling that approval could be granted to one institution, but revoked when that institution merges with another or transfers its planning approval to another institution.

The dominant nonprofit hospitals are often concerned with lessening the long-range planning advantage which is enjoyed by investor-owned hospital chains. Nonprofit hospitals are normally created when concerned citizens recognize that their community needs a hospital. That is, the hospital is planned after the need appears.

Investor-owned hospital chains, by contrast, are able to watch the movement of population and residential building permits. They can present a coherent defensible construction project to a community planning board before a single house is built. An extension of this planning advantage might mean that the investor-owned hospitals would come to dominate the growth areas of the countryside. Voluntary nonprofit hospitals would be left to enjoy the rotting urban core.

Another side of it is the questionable propriety of urban non-profit institutions buying out suburban profit-making ones with tax-free municipal bonds. When the profit-making hospital chains explain that they are selling out because state cost control regulation makes it impossible for them to survive financially, one has to wonder whether things are being squeezed a little.

One hears stories of planning agencies bargaining with hospitals: Merge with this one and we will let you build a new building, reduce your beds by fifty and you can have a certificate of need, don't buy a CAT Scanner with donated money or we might not let you expand your beds next time you ask. Since the life expectancy of the HSA depends on continued Congressional funding, the independence and impartiality of its judgments (or at least those of its salaried staff) will always be tempered by the prevailing political climate. Since the history of regulatory agencies is that they almost never save money and they almost always succumb to industry domination, one wonders if the two things are not the same thing. It may be difficult, but the hospitals will win. The revolving door of staff employment helps a little, too.

The HSA movement, perhaps echoing the consumer movement, has developed an alarmingly indiscriminate antitechnology bias. One could wish that the Swedes would hurry up and award the Nobel Prize to Hounsfield * for the CAT Scanner, thereby putting a stop to the current anti-CAT-scan nonsense. Somehow it has been overlooked that technology sometimes saves a lot of money (penicillin and polio vaccine) and sometimes costs a lot of money (cancer chemotherapy and respiratory inhalation therapy). But it has been stated with reasonable authority that the net effect of all technology advances of the past forty years has been to reduce costs.

Health benefits were even thrown in as a kicker, as they say in business. If you like, society could put technology on a zero balance cost budget, insisting that health care authorities fund expensive technology out of the profits from cost-saving technology.

So much for the HSA, and why the planning process isn't the right answer for the present boom in health costs, or even the

*On October 11, 1979, after this was written, it was announced that Godfrey Newbold Hounsfield of England and Allan McCleod Cormack of Massachusetts had been awarded the Nobel Prize for Medicine.—*Ed. Note.*

present boom in facility construction. Some anonymous delegate at the 1979 annual AMA convention rose to the microphone and remarked that it is very difficult to make an absolutely unique mistake, but that Congress has succeeded in doing so in two cases: Prohibition, and P.L. 93-641. What the situation needs is a medical Freddie Laker, not a medical United Nations.

Prospective Rate Control (Regulation by Imposed Nonmarket Incentives)

An inside joke in the regulatory field is that entry controls are redundant if you have rate control. That is, if you starve the industry to death you don't need to worry about any new firms trying to enter the field. As psychiatry professors emphasize that people always say exactly what they mean when they are joking, it doesn't pay to enjoy this joke too much if you ever expect to be sick.

Prospective rate control is price control. It is a method of imposing a fee schedule, as doctors would say in their own reimbursement system. A wide variety of formulas have been proposed for determining the fixed price which is set, and most systems introduce an appeals process for the hospitals to try to badger the fee up a little. A great deal of argument revolves around definitions of things, since switching the definition is a way of being paid a fee for a more complicated service than the one you performed. On the other hand, blind regulatory resistance at this point absolutely strangles innovation and progress. The word for this is public utility regulation, but price control is its essential feature.

Prospective rate setting is intended to give the hospital an incentive for efficiency which is not present in retrospective cost reimbursement. It has two hidden characteristics which are less laudable:

1. Those incentives are set by politicians.

2. The process continues to avoid the setting and payment of itemized charges.

The hidden characteristics reduce the marketplace to two teams of manipulative accountants, each trying to maximize his own set of subsidies. The regulator's accountant will be under pressure to maximize subsidies to political pressure groups, while the regulatee's accountant will be motivated to arrange subsidies for the most powerful pressure group in his institution at the moment. Sometimes the patients will benefit from the process, but that is accidental.

THREE TECHNICAL PROBLEMS WITH PROSPECTIVE RATE SETTING

The first technical problem grows out of the nonprofit nature of most hospitals. The hospital has an incentive to be more efficient because it will lose money if it is inefficient. But what does that mean? It would seem that losing money really just means that any such penalty is laid on the backs of (guess who?) the self-pay and commercially insured minority of patients. What is really created by suppressed costs is an incentive to get rid of complicated or expensive Medicaid or Medicare patients.[4] Some of the pending costs-control legislation in Washington proposes penalties for de- liberately altering case mix for this motive, but the impossibility of enforcement makes this provision almost laughable. Is it proposed that we forbid referral of complex cases to referral centers?

The second serious flaw in prospective rate setting is the present rapidity of change in the health care field. Regulation is a slow and cumbersome process which has fewest problems only when it is applied to industries which are changing very little, or very slowly in a predictable direction.

Since the reimbursement mechanism is pouring money into the health system, the health system is changing very rapidly. The only feasible regulatory response is to attempt to freeze the system into whatever pattern was contemplated by the regulatory design. The imposition of rigidities on a boiling health care system will either have tragic results for patients, or tragic results for politicians, or both.

The third problem is predicting in January what inflation will be next December.

THEORY OF THE HOSPITAL FIRM

It is amusing to read that the theory of the firm is not very far advanced in the case of hospitals. The translation of that jargon is

4. For the equivalent problem of physician fee schedules, consider Canadian medicine and shared health facilities. The response in both cases is the rejection of complex cases in favor of simple ones.

that it is hard to tell who is running the place and for what goals. So let's have a try at it, because new perceptions are apparently being sought.

The hospital prior to 1965 was dominated by the power groups who were essential to its function. The private patients were charged more than cost, to provide a surplus to the deficits of the ward service. If the surplus was inadequate, the balance was made up by donations. The doctors were important, because they brought in the private patients, and contributed their time for ward work and teaching. The donors and potential donors among the private patients were important. It was unusual for the break-even semiprivate patients to count for much, and the administrator was a significant factor only if he made himself so as a fund raiser or with visible administrative achievements.

Abruptly following 1965, there was very little charity, and there were droves of semiprivate patients. The doctors now became important if they brought in large numbers of semiprivate patients, otherwise not. The trustees were really no longer much use as fund raisers, although a trustee with political clout was nice. Consumer groups assert some right to be heard, but the plain fact is that they are free riders and the government is footing the bill. Let's face it, the golden rule prevails: The man with the gold makes the rules.

The curious thing is that the government has been so unaggressive in asserting *droit du seigneur* in this situation. It may possibly have to do with the fact that the 1979 HEW budget was larger than the gross national product of Great Britain, and indigestion is already acute. It may have to do with plans for retirement to a hospital job after one has one's federal pension vested. In any event, it is clear that the group closest to the federal fountain is best able to irrigate its own administrative garden.

THE FUTURE OF PROSPECTIVE RATE SETTING

Some future trends are safely predictable if we get into cost containment through prospective rate setting. The case mix of hospitals and the efficiency of patient flow can be adjusted to lengthen or shorten the average length of stay (in order to cause a decrease or increase in the *per diem* share of the total case cost) as needed. Costs can be overestimated and auditors will play fox and hounds trying to find the overestimate. Across-the-board slashes will be threatened or made, to flush out the Truth. Appeals will be made to politicians, and politians will be heard. Like retrospective cost-reimbursement, prospective cost setting is a system designed to force honest people to be manipulative in order to survive.

And a final horror is possible. Although existing studies suggest that prospective rate setting doesn't cut costs, it is just barely possible that it may cut costs as the system is refined. We would then have a system which was less costly than retrospective payment, but more expensive than market-determined pricing. Costs would inevitably fall in that range because the "profit" would be split between politically motivated subsidies and the bureaucratic subsidy of a small cost reduction to perpetuate the system.

Ask yourself whether rate control is necessary for Freddie Laker, and you see why rate control is wrong for hospitals.

The Rough Riders (Regulation by Antitrust Principles)

There are features of the health field which suggest to some the existence of monopoly. Monopoly is the special province of the Federal Trade Commission, and FTC members have been heard to grumble about it. The monopoly characteristics of the health field were almost invariably created by legislation, or at least by government. Regulation amounts to monopolistic behavior through the political process. But the Sherman Anti-trust Act was really designed to combat something else, called a "natural" monopoly.

The classical characteristics of a natural monopoly are that it:

1. Is the kind of business which enjoys unlimited "economies of scale." The bigger you are, the more advantage you have over competitors, so you get still bigger, if you are a natural monopoly.

2. Requires large amounts of seed capital to get started, so that new entrants have a lot to lose if they try to muscle their way into the field.

3. Is the kind of business where eventually the monopolist can raise prices as he pleases, with the result that the public receives no benefit from low costs. In the Clayton Antitrust Act, Congress later recognized that an entrenched monopolist can also unfairly lower prices to increase initial losses for new market entrants, who naturally have higher production costs.

The hospital field does not fit this pattern of a "natural monopoly," although it quite obviously has some appearances of monopoly. A similar paradox existed in the airline industry until the Carter administration put a stop to restricted route designation. Hire a couple of pilots, finance an airplane with an equipment mortgage, and hang out your shingle. As far as building a hospital is concerned, if you didn't understand Chapter 12, "Building Mrs. O'Leary's Hospital," just accept it on faith that it costs very little to build the biggest and best hospital you can design. No matter how empty it is, you are buffered against losses by retrospective cost-reimbursement.

So much for entry costs. What about economies of scale? In one sense, it doesn't matter because hardly any of your clients will be paying your charges. If you enlarge your viewpoint and regard the community at large or the government as your client, it is very difficult to be certain about economies in scale. On a theoretical level, it seems unlikely that a one-on-one service industry would have much scale economy. On an empirical level, however, it must be noticed that a great deal of concentration is taking place. It seems a possibility that the transformation of hospitals from labor-intensive to capital-intensive entities may eventually establish natural monopolies. At the moment, however, almost all of the monopoly characteristics of hospitals are strictly unnatural, created by governmental laws, licenses and regulations. Some of those are even desirable and necessary. But the patron saint of lower hospital costs is not Teddy Roosevelt, it's Freddie Laker.

---

*The big trouble with criticizing hospital expansion programs is that someone will think you favor the HSA entry limitation approach. And the big trouble with arguing for a market-determined price system is that someone else will think you are endorsing the crusade of the Federal Trade Commission for fair trade for limited-licenses practitioners. Freddie Laker is a great guy, but no one wants freedom from regulation to the point where planes are going to crash in the Atlantic.

22

A Meeting of the Rationing Board

It was twenty minutes past two, and the meeting had been called for two o'clock. The room was very quiet. The chairman tried very hard to look busy, looking through the papers in front of him. Each of the thirty places around the long mahogany table had a similar pile of papers, and fourteen of the members were seated in place, each behind a large white name card. Most of the members had accepted a cup of coffee from the staff, and a few were busy leafing through the papers. Several were chatting idly in low voices with their neighbors. Ten or twelve visitors and staff members were sitting in chairs around the wall. In the center of the table, but close to the place of the chairman was a tall stack of documents photocopied on pink paper—thirty bundles of ten pages, stapled together. Time passed. The chairman motioned to the chief staff assistant and asked him if he had called the absent members. The staff man nodded, raised his eyes to the ceiling, and shrugged his shoulders helplessly. The chairman was not pleased.

Through the door then walked a very tall man in a wrinkled blue suit who paused to look for his name on the cards at the table, then slipped into his designated seat. Dr. Bond. Although his entrance went largely unnoticed by the other board members, it instantly galvanized the chairman into animation, and eager smiles spread across the faces of the staff employees in the seats against the wall. Quorum. Now we can begin. The May 20th meeting of the ten-county regional Health Systems Agency was in session. The minutes of the previous meeting of the HSA were before everyone. Could we have motion for approval?

Most but not all of the board members broke off their conversations at the announcement of the chairman, turned themselves straight in their chairs and began hunting through the pile of papers at their places. When the minutes were located, the members began leafing through the stapled pages. "Mr. Chairman."

"Yes, Miss Gussy," said the chairman with a broad smile.

"I see that my name is not listed as present at the last meeting, which was the April 19th meeting. I'm sure I was here, and would like to have the secretary amend the minutes.

"Well, Miss Gussy, I don't want to dispute what you say, but I wonder if you aren't thinking of the *March* 19th meeting."

"Wasn't that the meeting when we talked about the St. Jerome Hospital fire sprinkler system? I remember very well being here."

"No, if you refer back in the minutes, you will see that the St. Jerome sprinkler matter was debated at the March 19th meeting. The April 19th meeting was adjourned early for lack of quorum. You weren't here, I'm sure, because Dr. Bond called for a quorum and we had to adjourn."

"Well, anyway, I just wanted . . ." began Miss Gussy, but she stopped abruptly as Dr. Bond stood up and leaned his long body across the table between her and the chairman, reached out the eraser end of a long yellow pencil, and snaked a stapled bundle of pink sheets off the top of the undistributed pile in front of the chairman.

Both the chairman and Miss Gussy were struck dumb by the sight of the pink paper being scooted over the table by the pencil. Dr. Bond captured his papers and settled back to read them. He placed the pink bundle on top of the other papers at his place, read the first page and the last page, and pushed his way through the middle pages with the rubber tip of the yellow pencil. Although every person at the table had fifty pages of reading material in front of him (or her), there was now no interest in looking at anything except the pink pages which Dr. Bond had. The chairman was particularly flustered to have it dramatized that he was holding something back for an opportune moment. For a full fifteen seconds the meeting sat in paralyzed silence watching Dr. Bond's pencil push through the packet. Although Dr. Bond ignored them all, it was he who broke the silence.

"Move approval of the minutes of the previous meeting."

The chairman reacted with gratitude that his meeting was back on the tracks, and asked if the motion was seconded. A dapper little man (Mr. Kiwanis) immediately next to the chairman seconded the motion. Mr. Kiwanis always seconded motions. When he occasionally found that he had seconded a preposterous motion, he rescued himself by saying that he had seconded it only to permit discussion to proceed. No one seemed to notice that Dr. Bond had not even glanced at the minutes he was moving to approve. No one except the chairman, who was in no position to draw attention to it.

"We have a number of very urgent matters on the agenda today," began the chairman, "so that we must proceed to item number one, which is the matter of the unauthorized CAT Scanner in Dr. Neurosurgeon's office."

"Mr. Chairman."

"Yes, Dr. Bond?"

"I believe that we previously agreed that the agenda, together with background material, would be sent out in advance of the meeting. A great many board members did not attend today, and some of the rest of us are rather slow readers."

"Dr. Bond, a quorum is present, as provided in the bylaws. And there are a number of staff employees present today who will be glad to supply any information the board might need. I think it is rather unfair to criticize the staff when they are working very hard to get the material here for the meetings. The mails are slow, you know."

"I see," said the old doctor. "And tell me just where the matter of the burn unit at Baptist Hospital can be found on the agenda? Or is the material on the pink sheet merely in preparation for next month's meeting, to save postage?"

"No, we are going to take that up this meeting. There is an urgent deadline for the HEW application, and we have to work against it. But that comes up later, and first we will take up the matter of the unauthorized CAT Scanner. I'm going to ask Mr. Jones of the staff to describe the problem."

While Mr. Jones was getting to his feet and arranging the flip charts for his presentation, every board member was shuffling through his pile of papers to find the material on the Baptist Hospital burn center. Gradually, the realization dawned on the members that the subject must be on the pink sheets, sitting so tantalizingly on the pile in the center of the table. But no one had the nerve to ask for a copy, since that would have been rude to Mr. Jones, who was straightening his shoulders for the big presentation on his subject of CAT Scanners.

"As you know," he began, "a CAT Scanner is an extremely expensive piece of equipment, averaging $300,000 apiece, and costing three hundred dollars every time it is used, that is, per usage unit. This HSA is on record as opposing the indiscriminate unnecessary proliferation of this new technology. There already is a CAT Scanner at the Baptist Hospital, only a twenty-minute drive from Dr. Neurosurgeon's office. It is for the board to decide, of course, but it is the very strong belief of staff that a second CAT Scanner would be an unnecessary and unjustified cost to the community." He sat down with a grim look on his face. The chairman had been whispering with the chief staff assistant, and was a little slow to follow up the presentation. Dr. Bond's voice cut in before the chairman could speak.

"Mr. Chairman, I believe I see Mr. O'Toole, the administrator of the Baptist Hospital in the audience, and Dr. Neurosurgeon is also here. Since Mr. O'Toole is a former employee of this HSA organization, perhaps he could tell us what his hospital's budget runs to."

O'Toole, who was busy preparing his remarks for the pink-pages item, rose uncertainly to his feet. "A hundred million dollars a year," he answered to no one in particular.

"Two million dollars a week," remarked Dr. Bond. "And you feel that a $300,000 machine would be too much competition for the community to endure? Perhaps it would be instructive to hear Dr. Neurosurgeon's point of view."

All heads turned toward the peppery little bald man who had been twisting and fidgeting in his chair against the wall. His lawyer sat next to him, and although the lawyer had been trying to persuade his client to let a lawyer do the talking, there was no stopping him. The chairman had not intended to recognize the doctor, but it did not matter. He was now talking loud and fast.

"Ladies and gentlemen, my big point is that I can save patients money, and save lots of money for Medicare, too. My partners and I will only charge a hundred dollars per examination, and you just heard that the hospital is charging three hundred. Let me just tell you how we can do it."

"These things cost $300,000, right?" he continued, with much waving of his hands. "The hospital is a nonprofit corporation, and doesn't pay taxes. But when my three partners and I buy the same equipment, we get a 10 percent equipment tax write-off, which is thirty thousand fewer dollars of income tax we have to pay. That's sixty thousand dollars worth of net income to someone in a 50 percent bracket. Then we depreciate the remaining $270,000 in five years, so the net cost to us is $105,000. So we can afford to perform the test for only a hundred dollars per exam. The machine only costs us a third of what it costs the hospital, so we only have to charge a third as much. Instead of holding me up, you ought to be closing down the three-hundred-dollar machine at the Baptist Hospital."

The chairman didn't understand all of that, and in any event wasn't listening very closely. After allowing Mr. O'Toole an opportunity to observe that the good doctor simply didn't understand the complexities of cost-reimbursement, he called for a vote. Eight to six opposed to Dr. Neurosurgeon's machine. Next item on the agenda . . . .

At that moment, an astonishing thing happened. A two-hundred-pound consumer representative in a scarlet dress stood up and noisily pulled back her chair at the table. While the whole room watched in shocked fascination, she climbed up on the chair and teetered unsteadily on her high heeled shoes, her large red garden hat flopping above the scene. When temporarily balanced, she spread her arms wide and bellowed, "Bullshit. Bullshit!" No one interrupted. "Don't talk about no 50 percent brackets. What I want to know is what you going to do for the poor people. Answer me that. What you going to do for the poor folks?"

At that, she came down from the chair, and in response to her wave, two other members of the board rose, and walked out of the room with her. The board sat in stunned silence as the footsteps were heard to go down the stairs.

"The meeting will come to order," said the chairman, looking ashen. "Staff will now distribute the pink sheets about the Baptist Hospital burn center."

"Mr. Chairman."

"Yes, Dr. Bond."

"I call for a quorum."

"Dr. Bond, Robert's *Rules of Order* state that if a quorum is present at the beginning of the meeting, the business may proceed."

"Well Mr. Chairman, I'm pretty sure the parliamentarian will find that both General Roberts and Mrs. Sturgis agree in their books that business may proceed only on a unanimous consent basis and that when any member makes a quorum call, the quorum must be present or the meeting must be adjourned."

"But, look, Dr. Bond, we will never be able to get our business done if . . . ."

"Mr. Chairman, I call for a quorum."

23

The Ownership Of Hospitals

Those who have thought hard about government regulation of all industries seem to agree that there is only one workable alternative: strengthening the marketplace. Those who prefer market-strengthening to regulation of medical care tend to urge health insurance modifications which require the patient to share his costs. The usual mechanisms are deductibles and co-payments. That approach appeals to me, too, and in the final chapter I propose some twists which might make deductions acceptable to their traditional opponent, organized labor.

However, it also seems to me that developing a stronger sense of prudence in the buyer of health care is not enough. We must also seek to induce more profit incentives in the seller of care, as well. Since non-profit institutions heavily predominate among hospitals, it is a matter of concern that their internal costs do not have the discipline of a profit motive. Never mind that it hurts the feelings of people to say so; complex organizations of two or three thousand employees need strong incentives to achieve maximum efficiency.

There are of course already a number of profit-making hospitals, and in some regions of the country they are flourishing. As mentioned earlier, they have done very well in anticipating the growth areas around the expanding urban rim. When they deal with Medicare, they are allowed to make a profit of about 6 percent on invested equity after taxes, and there are proposals with a good chance of passing through Congress which would allow them to close to 10 percent.[1]

1. The profit for investors in such hospitals is linked to the profit which the Government itself makes when it invests the reserves of the Social Security trust fund. The formula is that the investor-owned hospital may make a before-tax profit which is 1½ times the profit made by investment of the trust fund. After all, if you make equal profits by risking your money in a hospital or buying government bonds, you would buy bonds because they are safer. When this was written, the return was 8.4 percent. Corporate income tax then would cut this in half.

Unfortunately it is not easy for a voluntary hospital to change its corporate form to for-profit status in order to acquire extra Medicare payment. Governments do not extend tax exemptions willingly or without suspicion, and the laws are structured to prevent anyone from extracting profits from a tax-exempt organization by the process of selling or dissolving it. It seems very likely that direct conversion of non-profit hospitals to for-profit status would require enactment of special legislation. That proposed legislation would encounter the objection that profits for hospitals would directly cost Medicare more money, or patients more money, and the supposed later cost savings from enhanced efficiency would be unproven.

So it seems better to propose that the non-profit hospital retain its non-profit status, but spin off a for-profit subsidiary corporation, wholly owned by the non-profit parent. I am not a lawyer, but I know of non-profit corporations which own profit-making subsidiaries, so it seems to be possible to do it. Perhaps a good way of thinking of the arrangement would be to suggest that the common stock of the subsidiary corporation would be part of the investment portfolio of the endowment fund of the non-profit owner.

It occurs to me that a useful psychological transformation might take place if two corporate boards of directors and two teams of management evolved out of this spin-off process. The two boards would have to exist "on paper" anyway, so is it possible that temperment and incentive would lead the board of the new subsidiary to drive hard for its mission of business-like efficiency and profit, while the board of the non-profit owner would add the role of restraining anti-social aggressiveness in the subsidiary to its main role of conducting teaching, research, and charitable activities? The evolving attitudes of the ambivalent non-profit board would be a fascinating sociological study. Their mission is charity; their income comes from tough business practice. One would hope that the formalization of the whole non-profit hospital paradox in their meetings would eventually spread out and ultimately clarify American society's goals about the same subjects.

Since it would be absolutely unacceptable to force our most prestigious institutions into changing to for-profit incorporation against their will, incentives must be considered. The Medicare profit allowance has existed for years, without causing a stampede toward investor ownership. Perhaps we can achieve two goals for cost containment at the same time. Is it possible that Congress could be persuaded to replace retrospective cost reimbursement with payment of posted charges, but only on condition that a for-profit subsidiary is created? One would suppose this might be justified somewhat in the mind of Congress by the reflection that much of the difference between cost and charge would immediately return as corporate income tax. The process might be described as the isolation of the charitable function from the taxable function. The incentive might be described as a return to fair market pricing.

It is hard to imagine that non-profit hospitals could blithely ignore the alternative incentives of profit on cost-reimbursed income or profit margin on posted charge payments. One would hope that the latter alternative would be the preferred option. It would seem entirely legitimate to refuse to pay the higher posted charges to any hospitals which declined to pay taxes on the resulting profits, so unfair discrimination should not be an issue.

One last incentive could be offered to hospitals which agreed to separate formally the charitable and business functions. It grows naturally out of the act of creating a new corporation, because there is a big problem to be coped with.

It is rather late in the book to be introducing a major new problem, and we really aren't. It was latent in the first chapter, when Mr. O'Toole and Mrs. O'Leary were planning big things. You will recall that she was very excited about the possibility of unlimited borrowing, followed by tax-exempt investment. It isn't quite that easy, but there is something to it.

Let us go back to Mrs. O'Leary, and postulate four different scenarios for a contribution by her of a million dollars for a million-dollar hospital building.

> SCENARIO ONE: She makes the million-dollar contribution and a million-dollar building is built. *Outcome:* At the end of forty years, the depreciation payments restore a million dollars cash to the hospital. The profit is the salvage value of the building at that time. (We are simplifying, of course.)

> SCENARIO TWO: She gives the million dollars, but plans change and no building is erected. The money is invested. *Outcome:* Ignoring inflation and fluctuations of investments,

the money could earn ten percent interest, compounded. Since money at ten percent doubles every seven years, the hospital might have approximately $50 million at the end of forty years. Even 7 percent would lead to $16 million.

SCENARIO THREE: She decides not to give the money after all. The hospital goes ahead and builds the building by borrowing money and repaying the loan through the reimbursement mechanism. *Outcome:* At the end of the forty years, the hospital has acquired the salvage value of the building with no investment of its own. If it is in for-profit status, it would have earned profits during the forty-year use of the building by treating patients.

SCENARIO FOUR: She gives the money, but the hospital invests it as an endowment. At the same time, the building is built with borrowed money. *Outcome:* It definitely is *not* true that the hospital at forty years has both $50 million and the salvage value. The rules of cost-reimbursement agencies require that interest payments be first offset against investment income. If the interest on the loan is greater than the endowment return, the net interest excess is reimbursable. In that case, the hospital ends up with Mrs. O'Leary's million dollars, plus the salvage value of the structure. On the other hand, if the interest cost is less than endowment income, the difference compounds for forty years and is added to the salvage value.[2]

A main lesson to be learned is that investment of the endowment provides an overwhelmingly greater source of funds for teaching, charity, and research than putting the money into bricks and mortar. Or, to put it another way, it is so disadvantageous to charitable functions to build a building that there must be an overwhelming need for a new building before it should be even considered by a hospital with an endowment.

A hospital without endowment has no such restraint placed upon

2. It becomes apparent that the low interest rates which characterize tax-exempt municipal bonds make an important advantage for that lending mechanism, which must be set against the greater financial latitude sometimes enjoyed by a conventional mortgage with a friendly bank.

it, and there really is an inequity in the situation. An accounting rule, intended to prevent speculation with borrowed money, ends up penalizing charitable contributions, thus differentially penalizing a hospital which in somebody's opinion was worthy of reward. The only good thing which can be said about this situation is that it does create an incentive to a hospital with endowment to invest it instead of using it for building enhanced structures.

If we persuaded hospitals to split the charitable and business functions into two corporations, this problem would become a severe one. Is it fair to let the charitable corporation invest while the business corporation borrows? On the other hand, is it fair to prevent it? One can easily see why the reimbursement agencies moved to restrain the dual process of borrowing and investing, but they are possibly preventing something which is not inherently wrong. They are illustrating the fact that the cost-reimbursement system, whether retrospective or prospective, regulated or free, is a system which relentlessly searches out ways to pose unexpected problems.

It seems very hard to believe that Congress would permit simultaneous borrowing and investing without exacting a price in return, since the dual process is more commonly known as investing on margin. Margin accounts are a severely regulated activity, even when the government has neither provided nor tax-sheltered any of the investor's funds.

Since it is a foregone conclusion that this matter would get Congressional scrutiny if the two-corporation system became popular, it is only right that the rules be defined before any hospital is asked to get into the situation. They might as well be defined in a way that gives an incentive to minimize costs and maximize charity.[3]

---

3. A related issue is the buying and selling of hospitals, since purchase and sale is a way of separating corporations. A hospital that had no endowment when it built its building can be acquired by another which has an endowment. A large number of variations of this theme can be imagined, and many of them can be imagined to be inequitable.

24

Health Catastrophe
Insurance: Catastrophe for
Whom?

One of the things I have learned in writing this book is that it takes six months between the time an author surrenders his manuscript to the publisher and the first moment when the public can read what he has to say. This normal minimum time lag (a full year is more typical) means that public awareness of the issues being debated in Congress depends on newspapers, television, and magazines, all of whom by their nature have to produce information which is summarized, hence lacking in comprehensiveness. For this reason, the legislative process is a slow one, having to wait for public opinion to coalesce. Meanwhile, authors hesitate to write books about pending legislative proposals, because the issue may have come and gone before the book reaches its audience.

At the time this book goes to press, there are three major pieces of health insurance legislation pending in Congress, ready to start their painful amendment progress through committees, passing with new amendments through first one and then the other side of Congress, working through compromises in a joint House-Senate conference committee, and then being signed or vetoed by the President. Since there is no way of predicting the status of things when the reader gets this book, it is necessary to discuss only principles involved rather than specific details.

Senator Russell Long of Louisiana has proposed a bill which would establish a national system of insurance covering those infrequent but disastrous situations in which the patient develops an illness so severe that the costs are themselves a catastrophe to his family.

As a nation, we cringe at the idea that someone might be placed in the position where his medical survival either is abandoned for reasons of cost or results in the impoverishment of his whole family. During the Great Depression of the 1930s, there were real instances of men throwing themselves out skyscraper windows so their families could collect life insurance; society was shocked when it happened, but society could sympathize with the motives of self-sacrifice. Insurance against health cost catastrophes has great public appeal.

It is also fairly cheap. We hear that Senator Long's bill would add a cost of about $6 billion to the present $192 billion national health care budget, if a health catastrophe is defined as one which has more than a threshold cost of $3,500. The extra federal cost of Senator Long's proposal would be about 3 percent. Even our shaky national economy and our internationally weakened dollar might be able to absorb such a cost for such a national aspiration.

President Carter has made a proposal (the Ribicoff-Rangel bill) which includes health catastrophe coverage, and adds a consolidation of Medicare and Medicaid.[1] Senator Kennedy proposes comprehensive national health insurance including coverage of health catastrophes, plus prospective rate setting,[2] plus a financing mechanism based on graduated progressive taxation rather than risk experience-adjusting. All three bills thus have the common denominator of health catastrophe coverage. In a national election year, national health catastrophe insurance could well become law.

The first thing to notice about health catastrophe insurance is that it really is insurance. While catastrophic costs apparently amount to 3 percent of total health care costs, nothing like 3 percent of the population is at risk of having such a catastrophe. Each such occurrence is so expensive that the number of people to whom it happens is much less than one in thirty; consequently, even a wealthy family would regard the small premium as well worth paying and be glad they mostly never needed to use it. All the rest of what we call health insurance is really just prepayment; we do expect to spend the money some day. Prepayment is a large Christmas savings fund, which on average is renewed every seven years.

It thus develops that we must consider what would happen to

1. See Chapter 16, "The New Poor."
2. See Chapter 21, "Regulation: Better is Not Always Best."

the pre-payment mechanism if all Americans were really insured against serious health costs. The sum of $3,500 is only half of the cost of a new automobile, but even $500 is a financial blow to the majority of people, especially young people with overextended credit. Furthermore, we have grown accustomed to the pre-paid mechanism, have adjusted our personal finances to assume its presence, and are timid and conservative about change. So it might be a long time before very many people got up their nerve to drop the pre-paid premium and set aside $3,500 internally in their personal savings for use (with interest earned) as self-insurance.

But let us try to imagine the alternatives these people would find if they considered it. Self-insurance[3] has growing popularity among employer groups, and even national governments,[4] since it cuts out the (appreciable) costs of the middleman. Self-insurance for individuals would be equally attractive for individuals, and the health catastrophe coverage would serve the role of high-risk reinsurance. Maybe we're getting somewhere.

Health catastrophe insurance is already available as something you can buy. It really is nothing but a high-deductible, very generous health insurance plan which presupposes no "basic" coverage. The unfortunate insurance term for such a policy is uncoordinated excess medical coverage.[5] While I am in no position to make national actuarial projections, some idea of the cost of such health insurance alternatives is available to me in the group health insurance plans offered to the Philadelphia County Medical Society for its members. Several similar proposals have come to me as advertising mail, so it seems possibly representative to look at this example which extends coverage up to a million dollars per lifetime. The members, for whom no underlying basic prepaid health insurance is assumed, have their choice of four annual deductible levels, at four different premiums. They also have a choice of conventional pre-paid first-dollar coverage through Blue Cross and Blue Shield, which is included in the following table as if it were health coverage with a zero deductible.

3. See chapters 14 and 15 "The Moral Hazard of Third & Fourth Parties," and "Sticky Wicket."
4. See Chapter 19, "Canadian Medicine: A Fly Caught In The Amber."
5. It is appalling that a sales industry which puts such emphasis on public image would employ such an invidious title for a product. How about calling it "basic medical disaster protection," for instance?

DEDUCTIBLE	ANNUAL PREMIUM
None (Blue Cross plus Blue Shield)	$1735.56[6]
$500 Deductible (up to $1 million)	1070.64
$1000 Deductible (up to $1 million)	728.28
$5000 Deductible (up to $1 million)	279.30
$25,000 Deductible (up to $1 million)	61.50

One must be careful of extrapolating from the premiums of one small group to the whole nation, proposing to make national policy. Our members may have coordinated dual coverage, they may be entitled to professional discounts, and they may have an unusual health pattern. But the magnitude of the figures allows considerable latitude for the basic conclusion: You save a pile of money by eliminating first-dollar coverage.

Let's play games with the numbers, just to emphasize them. Suppose you took out the $1,000 deductible policy and were lucky enough to stay well for twenty years; with compound interest you would have saved $25,000. You could then afford to drop your premium to $61.50 per year, and you would be earning $2,500 per year interest on your savings in the savings bank. Or, one could easily imagine a progressive system in which you start out with a $500 deductible policy, and if you remain healthy you can later afford to drop down to a $1,000 deductible. If you still are lucky, in a few years you can afford a $5,000 deductible; and a few years later you can afford the $25,000 deductible. The joke is that at that point, you could afford full first-dollar coverage, since the investment interest would pay for it into perpetuity.

Now, take it slowly. This is a pretty sophisticated concept, radically at variance with existing habits and attitudes. No one should expect a national stampede to drop prepaid "insurance" just because real insurance is available, even universally mandated. But the idea is there, and two hundred million Americans use many different approaches to things; everybody likes to save

6. Blue Cross Co-Pay comprehensive (1095.00), Blue Shield Prevailing Fee (640.56). To be absolutely comparable in benefits, one might have to take out the $5,000 deductible in addition; perhaps the $25,000 deduction would suffice. It probably is an important hidden perplexity that a great many people who are covered by Major Medical policies fail to submit claims which would be covered. This unexpected source of profitability for the insurance company probably grows out of the fact that benefits are negotiated for groups by their employers or unions, and the beneficiaries are largely unaware of what coverage they actually have.

money. It seems entirely possible that the pioneer members of the community, plus the improvident ones who are careless about insurance anyway, might start a gradually widening spiral of self-insurance which might become pretty popular pretty fast. Most people would probably hang on to their first-dollar coverage for a year to see if all this was for real, but an idea that could save 10 percent of income might travel pretty fast. The only people who would have a clear financial incentive to retain their first-dollar coverage would be the ones who know they are sick, or those who are planning to have babies. The existing first-dollar policies would be pushed into adverse selection of risks, the premiums would go up fast, and more people would drop out. Guess who would have an incentive to try to prevent all this? In addition to the insurance carriers who would be dismayed to see their businesses destroyed, the people who had paid premiums for years but were now facing illness expense would have a legitimate complaint. The imposition of compulsory health catastrophe insurance would require a seven-year phase-out fund to prevent such inequities, although the resulting national savings would probably easily justify it.

Look at what else might happen. If a large number of people were self-insured for most medical expenses, they would pay posted hospital charges [7] instead of having calculated costs paid to the hospital. This would broaden the base of charge-paying clients for each hospital, and therefore the markup between costs and charges would narrow. Not only would moral hazard [8] be reduced, but posted charges could be reduced, and the medical component of the cost of living index would be reduced [7] closer to true expenditures. Maybe we could think of phasing out cost-reimbursement entirely,[9] and then Senator Long might be eligible for sainthood.

Politics must be considered. In the first place, Senator Kennedy and other proponents of extending "comprehensive" first-dollar coverage would feel pressed to head off such a threat to their proposals. But it is said that the principal force urging these proponents on to comprehensive first-dollar benefits is organized labor. The key to achieving a workable compromise is to offer something to labor.

7. See Chapter 7, "A Primer From the Trustees."
8. See Chapter 21, "Why Do Hospitals Cost So Much?"
9. See Chapter 8, "Further Subsidies."

If the reader will have a little patience with numbers, our example of the various deductible premiums now commercially available may illustrate something else. Our problem, remember, is that health insurance fringe benefits are now a part of the worker's income. Naturally, he doesn't want to see his income reduced, and he may even be sophisticated enough to resist the imposition of income tax on his present tax-shelter. So, as part of our bargaining, why don't we offer to pay the worker his deductible portion in extra cash, and give him a tax exemption for it? Looked at from his employer's point of view, the resulting wage cost we could be talking about would be the sum of the cash deductible payment plus the cost of the insurance premium. When the employer does his sums, he might well find that the new package could cost less than the old one.

PLAN	COST TO EMPLOYER
	(deductible plus premium)
First Dollar Coverage	$ 1,735.56
$500 Deductible	1,570.64
$1000 Deductible	1,728.28
$5,000 Deductible	5,279.30
$25,000 Deductible	$25,061.50

It can be seen that while the employee has an incentive to have the deductible go as high as possible, the employer has an incentive to have it be somewhere around $500. So, a bargain might be struck at $700 deductible, and the next year the negotiating team could look at the figures to find the most advantageous new deductible which both sides would be seeking. A market mechanism might just emerge, and such self-correcting systems are greatly to be desired.

Would a deductible of $500 to $700 achieve the same result as a $3,500 deductible? Yes, and it might soften some of the disruptions that we imagined might result from a shift to self-insurance. A $500 deductible would be high enough to strengthen the medical marketplace, because most people spend less than that much in an average year, and most doctors obtain the majority of their income from patients whose total yearly medical expenditure is less than a $500 deductible. Furthermore, those patients who spend more than $500 are mostly receiving services which are the same services as the low-cost patients get, so the market mechanism would still legitimize the fees. It is true that some services like heart surgery would probably invariably cost more than the deductible threshold and hence be immune to market-set pricing. For services of that type, a relative-value system would have to be employed in which an above-threshold fee was determined to be worth a certain multiple of market-set fees. Never mind that the Federal Trade Commission presently opposes relative value pricing. The FTC was created by Congress, and if Congress wants a relative-value system, that ends the matter.

It would be interesting to see how the leadership of organized labor would react to this proposal. Some say that they would be concerned that some of their members might later suffer from their own improvidence if they ever got their hands on the cash, using it to pay debts instead of medical bills (you can see from the lingo that I have talked to some of them). But it is possible that they feel trapped in old slogans, realize that paternalism is a little out-dated for adults making $11 an hour ($22,000 a year) in 1979. The longshoremen are paid over $6 an hour in fringe benefits alone, and doubtless the membership would enjoy seeing some of that in the pay packet. Maybe the union leadership would like to change their traditional posture, and secretly wouldn't mind losing a few of these arguments. It seems worth exploring.

But before we sell health catastrophe insurance like snake oil, let's look at two major problems with it. The biggest problem is the obvious one of unlimited cost overruns. You could say that catastrophic coverage amounts to proclaiming we won't pay for it unless it is expensive. Guess what, things just might get expensive. The chronic renal dialysis program will cost over $1 billion next year, for forty thousand patients. I have been to security analysts' meetings in which the technology manufacturing industry was licking its chops in anticipation of national health insurance of any variety.

Senator Kennedy has a proposed remedy for that, called prospective rate control, but called rationing by me. You would have thought we all would have learned something from the Volstead Act, but apparently we might yet again be doomed to repeat the mistakes of history just because the term prospective rate control sounds so obscure. My own feeling is that the great majority of services which would qualify as a financial catastrophe over $3,500 would consist simply of a large volume of the same services which would have had their prices set by the market below $500 per year, if we could simply get rid of first-dollar coverage. Relative-value pricing would do the rest, if it became clear that there were significant abuses. Finally, it would seem to be a prudent safeguard to keep this insurance in the private sector, where the insurance companies would be able to withdraw from the market if costs got out of hand. It would be in everyone's interest to prevent things from reaching that point; but if they did, at least the cost overrun should not be allowed to get linked to the printing presses of the Treasury's Bureau of Printing and Engraving. There would surely be an enormous fuss if health insurance carriers refused to continue in the business, but at least they could be counted on to face facts. A federalized health insurance plan might well be unable to face the political heat that it had failed, and national inflationary consequences might be tragic. What politician in England would dare propose that the British Health Service should be abandoned? But still, in July, 1979, the British plumbers' union included private health insurance in their wage package, and that's as clear a sign of failure of the National Service as you could imagine.

The other problem with health catastrophe insurance is the possibility that it may be difficult to distinguish health cost catastrophes from chronic custodial care. Being old and senile is a catastrophe, all right, but it isn't what you can pay for with $6 billion. This one isn't an easy issue. Senile people get sick, and sick people get senile.

Since the country hasn't made up its mind about coping with this major coming problem, it is not expected to approve of sneaking it in through the back door of health catastrophes.

So health catastrophe insurance all in all may not be a bad idea, and with some clear thinking and clever modification it might just become splendid. It still suffers from the central problem of finding a way to confine the definition of a health catastrophe to what we now understand it to be, and avoiding the warping of the concept into a bandwagon for everything else to climb aboard. This might be a reasonable thing for the PSRO system to be asked to address, although it would need time to achieve an answer.

All in all, though, it looks a lot safer to try this idea out in the private insurance industry before we lock it into place nationally. Maybe all it needs is salesmanship, but probably it needs to prove itself. The accommodation of truly poor people obviously is a separate problem.

I guess there is one more problem. If all the dreams came true, and by using high-deductible insurance the whole pre-payment health system developed market-based pricing, and cost-reimbursement became ancient history, and the financing mechanism stopped twisting medical care into a pretzel, our hospitals would then probably start to look a little tacky, and the doctors would then have a few more bad debts to write off. But that would seem a very small price to pay for a very narrow escape from catastrophe.

25

The Cost of Insurance Moral Hazard: Whose Cost?

It's possible that the other chapters of this book have so implacably illustrated the evils of overinsuring health costs that the reader may think I am saying that nearly all health costs are already insured. That is only true of hospital costs, and for that reason the hospital has provided the most painful examples of the corrupting effects of release from marketplace discipline. The summer 1979 issue of *HCFA* (Health Care Financing Administration) *Review* conveniently provides the information that 33 percent of all personal health expenditures really were paid out-of-pocket in America in 1978. The total was $55.3 billion.

When anyone speaks of "comprehensive" national health insurance, he means that most or all of that $55.3 billion should be paid through the insurance mechanism instead of out-of-pocket. If the phraseology is "universal" health insurance, it is intended that another $45.4 billion (26 percent) which is covered by private health insurance should be absorbed by government reimbursement, as the Canadians have done. When the talk is of "uniform consolidation of government-financed health costs," it is intended that another $18.5 billion now provided by state and local governments would become a federal responsibility. This all amounts to quite a lot of billions.

Let's try a score card of the current Congressional proposals, reducing the dollars to percentages of our national health bill to make things a little simpler.

The present federal share is 28 percent.

Senator Long's Health Catastrophe Insurance would add 3 percent, making the federal share 31 percent.

President Carter's proposal would add the state share of Medicaid funds, bringing the federal share to 41 percent.

Senator Kennedy's comprehensive proposal would surely end up with some exclusions, but at least in theory it might go up to 74 percent. While the bill's language suggests that the other 26 percent would remain with private insurers, there is significant sentiment that a feature called "pooling of premiums" process is nothing but a bureaucracy in disguise, and would bring the federal share the rest of the way to 100 percent.

A range from 28- to 100-percent control of the finances (and shortly thereafter the policies) of the second largest industry in the nation is quite a reach. Since the benefits of permitting this to happen are obscure to me, I shall leave its defense to its proponents. Let's look at its cost.

The insurance mechanism is not cheap. It gets more expensive as the average size of the claim gets smaller. Medicare is divided into Part A, which pays hospitals, and Part B, which pays doctors. The *HCFA Forum* reports that the administrative costs of running Part A are 2 percent of the claims cost, while Part B costs 7.5 percent of the claims cost for administration. The difference reflects the larger size of the average hospital bill compared with the average doctor bill. It seems reasonable to suppose that the administrative overhead cost for paying for prescription drugs through the insurance mechanism would be even more expensive. In fact, these global averages surely obscure the fact that many covered claims are already too small to justify the use of anything but cash payments. Does it make sense to add an average claims-payment cost of $6 to a $10 service? What do you suppose a druggist would say if you asked him to mail you a bill for a toothbrush? Or if you offered to give him a personal check to pay for one aspirin tablet?

Think of all the medical things you now pay cash for, and ask whether the insurance claims cost of $6 to $9 would be justified by them. To help your contemplation, here is a partial list:

• Routine office visits
• Prescription drugs
• Unlimited psychiatric treatment

- Eyeglasses
- Nursing home care
- False teeth
- Routine immunizations
- Weight reduction
- Hypnosis to stop smoking
- Cosmetic surgery
- Genetic counseling
- Geriatric day care centers
- Education for self-care
- Marriage counseling
- Sex education
- Laxatives
- Sunglasses
- Preretirement counseling
- Helicopter ambulance services
- Treadmill monitoring of joggers
- Contact lenses

In 1978, the total cost of prepayment and insurance administration for health costs was $10 billion. While that only represents 5 percent of the national health budget of $192.4 billion, it represents 10 percent of the $100.4 billion of prepaid and insured personal health expenditures. If the insurance mechanism were extended into all of the nickel-and-dime bills of the present out-of-pocket portion of health costs, the administrative overhead costs would definitely go up. If we were careless about the benefits we gave out, the claims processing costs would be a scandal.

Now, as a provider of care, I am acutely aware that my secretary and I are fillers-out of insurance forms. We can't bill people for preparing insurance forms, at least not most of them, so this cost of insurance is shifted over to the fee as part of overhead. By this system, the insurance mechanism seems to be a lot cheaper than it really is, and the 2 percent Medicare Part A administrative cost is a good example of it. What do you suppose those hospital clerks and computer operators are doing with most of their time? Performing the hidden administrative costs of Blue Cross, Medicare, and Medicaid, that's what. Let's add 3 percent for this hidden cost of insurance.

But we've only begun to total up the cost of health insurance; 13

percent is just the beginning. There is the hidden interest cost. You lose interest on your money two ways with insurance: on the way in, and on the way out. If you should draw money out of a savings account to pay your health insurance premium, you would see a good illustration that it costs you interest to buy insurance rather than self-insure. And, on the other end, if you had to borrow money while you waited for the insurance check to be paid to you, you would become aware that there is interest on the floating money which someone gets, and someone else loses out on. Such interest income is a very important part of the financing of insurance. Almost all casualty insurance companies pay out as much in claims as they collect in premiums; their profits come from investment of their reserves (i.e., your money). I have been told by actuaries that a malpractice insurance company can break even if its claims are 117 percent of its premiums, since there is a particularly long delay between occurrences and final settlement. All of these examples are intended to show that the insurance system is costing the premium-paying subscriber a price which he does not realize he is paying in forgoing the opportunity to make interest on his own money. It would be my feeling that it is conservative to assign a 3.5 percent cost to the health insurance mechanism for this purpose, (2.5 percent on the premium, 1.0 percent on the delay in claims processing). We're now up to 16.5 percent as an average cost of the health insurance mechanism, and there's more to come.

Let's look at a little thing called errors. Obviously, there are errors in the insurance company's favor, and errors in favor of subscribers and providers. But the human tendency is to complain more about errors that go against you than to challenge an error in your favor. So the net effect of errors is to add another 1.5 percent cost to the insurance mechanism. Listen to what the director of HCFA's Office of Policy and Program Development had to say about errors in the Medicaid program:[1]

> In the AFDC program in 1973, the national payment error rate was 16 percent. Many states launched a rigorous error reduction program, and by June, 1976, the national error rate had been reduced to 8.5 percent. . . .

1. HCFA *Forum*—Vol. 2, No. 5, 1978, p. 30.

As the Medicaid program continued to grow, the dollar losses due to eligibility errors have increased to near-staggering levels. HCFA calculates that in fiscal year 1977, more than $1.1 billion in federal and state dollars were paid for medical services for ineligible persons.

HEW investigators indicate that another $600 million of Medicaid funds was paid out needlessly; the beneficiaries actually were covered by some other form of insurance. An additional $200 million was lost due to claims-processing errors. Thus, the total loss for fiscal year 1977 is estimated at nearly $2 billion. If this growth in erroneous payments continues, the picture for fiscal year 1981 could show a cumulative total of more than $10 billion needlessly spent.

Well, we've now got up to 18 percent as a conservative cost of the health insurance mechanism. We haven't counted the 12 percent loss due to eligibility determination and failure to subrogate, because we're totalling up the cost of comprehensive universal health insurance, which would presumably include everybody and exclude other insurance. We estimate the cost of using pre-paid insurance as at least 18 percent, without even considering the really expensive feature of it, which is the moral hazard that people will take a free ride, and the linked cost of trying to police the system to prevent people from taking appreciably more advantage of the system than the prevailing normative amount. If you assign a cost of insurance moral hazard which is equal to the increase in medical costs above the rise in the cost of living, in my opinion you won't be far wrong. Eliminate all of this cost of the insurance mechanism, and with the savings you could then make all medical care totally free every fourth year. Let's be sure to make that be election year; sort of like feeding the lions when they are most dangerously hungry.

26

The Descent into the Lower World

Two doctors walked down the stone stairs from the first floor of the hospital, turned on the landing, and continued down the rest of the stairs to the basement. The tall man with the white hair walked slightly ahead, and seemed to be more certain of where he was going than the young woman intern. A stethoscope and notebooks bulged out of the pockets of her jacket and flopped awkwardly as she walked. They paused in a corridor of blank unmarked doors.

"It's the second door," the man said, and the young woman moved quickly forward to open it. It was always uncertain whether age should resist habit and precede beauty. Both of them recognized that for the moment the role of age was uncongenial to him and of beauty uncongenial to her. So she pushed ahead.

"The door is locked," she said, "maybe we should call and see if it's postponed." Without replying, the older doctor moved forward to push a button and a bell rang loudly. The door was cautiously opened by a large black man in a white uniform, who threw it wide when he saw who was there.

"Hello, Opol, how are you? Go ahead in Sybil." The two entered a large, brightly lit laboratory, whose principal feature was an extremely large stainless steel worktable to which were attached numerous hoses and utility outlets. Another gray-haired man with dark horn-rimmed glasses was in the room. He wore a large rubber apron. On seeing the visitors, the man in the apron ignored the girl, and flashed a smile to the other man. "Welcome." The newcomer smiled warmly in return and said, "Hi Jerry. Yes, I have the postpermission. How is it that the boss himself is working on a Saturday morning?"

In what was meant as a pleasant joshing, the man in the apron turned toward the young woman and said pointedly, "The younger generation in my department don't show the same diligence that is displayed by house officers of the Department of Medicine." The young woman kept a perfectly blank face, so he turned away and said, "Shall we begin?"

"Yes. My patient was ninety-one years old and I'm pretty sure she had coarctation of the aorta."

"No surgery?"

"No. No nothing. So far as I know, this is the longest survival on record." At this point, the young woman interrupted.

"I'm very sorry, but I have to leave," she said, "I'll check back later." The two older men turned to look at her, but she was out the door.

"Well, don't worry about it. In our day we didn't have any money to go anywhere on our weekends off. So we had to hang around the hospital." The two men fell easily into conversation even though they had only fleetingly seen each other in recent years. But they had thirty years of shared experiences, firmly based on three years of close companionship at the beginning. "It looks as though she was born with a coarctation. To live to be ninety-one with that is remarkable."

"She used to be a patient of Perry MacNeal's. When he turned her over to me he made her promise to give me postpermission. She told me he said, 'Your body belongs to Dr. Aeneas, but your heart belongs to me!' And I'm very sure that's what he said, because no one else on earth could have said it."

"That's pretty good. There are some gallstones, here. Did she have a sense of humor, or was she mad about his lack of respect for a dowager?"

"She thought it was hilarious. I always enjoyed her visits. She was a dancer in Ziegfield's Follies, and hung around the advertising and show biz crowd even after she was eighty. I'm sure you've met her type. They dominate conversation by calling every spade a damned shovel. Speaking of Perry, he made a crack the other day. 'We used to make rounds with the interns and residents to teach them how to practice medicine,' he said, 'but nowadays we make rounds with interns and residents to teach them how *not* to practice medicine.' "

"You clinicians are having a hard time learning to teach with private patients, aren't you?" asked the pathologist. "I don't see why everyone is in such a hurry to exercise responsibility. Responsibility is what you get in great excess once you finish your training, and you're stuck with it the rest of your life."

"Yes, well, our problems on the medical service involve just the scufflings of egotists. Nothing serious. What I don't understand though is how anybody is going to learn to do surgery when the patients are all private patients. Imagine a scared girl who is delivering her first baby allowing the resident to deliver it. Particularly when her insurance entitles her to have the chief of obstetrics, and the chief of obstetrics is standing right there. There seems to be some hemorrhagic cystitis, doesn't there?"

"That's from your catheter. They all have it, these days. You may have saved her once, but sooner or later they all come to an illness you can't save them from. So then they come visit us here in the basement where their expenses look pretty futile."

"You know, I've wondered whether we couldn't devise a system of matching illnesses with subsequent longevity, through the Social Security number."

"What do you mean?"

"Well, the Social Security system sends everybody a check every month, but it is supposed to stop when the client dies. You could just imagine all those checks going to mail boxes forevermore unless they made an effort to trace deaths and stop sending the checks."

"Yes, I agree, but I don't follow you."

"If you know that a thousand dollars was spent on a certain case of pneumonia on a certain date, you need to know a second date, the date of later death. If the interval between spending the money and date of death was a thousand days, three years, then it cost a dollar a day to save her life from pneumonia. Conversely, if you spend a thousand dollars on day one, and date of death is day two, then it cost a thousand dollars a day to treat that situation. You can form your own opinion of the quality of that day."

"I see. And your idea is that every time a surgeon removes a cancer, the date is recorded. When that patient's Social Security number comes up on purge in the computer system, you can do the calculating of cost per day saved. Am I right?"

"Very right. You would have to safeguard confidentiality, but I really don't think it can be claimed that you have a right to privacy about the fact of your own death. The person who was doing the study would have to establish his right to possess the Social Security number and the medical facts. But his right to obtain that last bit, the vital statistic of death, seems to be clear enough. If the computer started to show that people under one kind of therapy weren't living for as many days as people given a different therapy, then maybe we would have a rapid way of picking up unsuspected toxicity of a new drug."

"That's quite an idea. Every time the pathology department made a diagnosis of cancer, we could add the patient's Social Security number to our files and then, when we wanted to know how long the patient eventually lived, we could just get the number out and ask Social Security if he were still alive. It would sort of be like the Golden Bough of the Aeneid, a preauthorization that you had a right to invade the kingdom of the dead and describe what you found."

"That's the point. Since all you want is the date of death, there really should be no confidentiality problem. The date isn't any good to you unless you know something else about the patient. The time to insist on confidentiality is when you are getting the original information."

"Give me an example."

"Well, suppose you had a new experimental drug. You would ask the patient to agree to give you his Social Security number and permission to inquire periodically about his health. If people who took the drug began to appear on the death list sooner than their life expectancy, you would begin to wonder if the drug had unsuspected toxicity."

"Wait a minute. If you did that with everyone who went into an oxygen tent, you would soon conclude that oxygen tents were killing people. After all, you don't get oxygen unless you are very sick to begin with."

"Of course that's true. You can only use this approach on drug therapy if you have another group of people with the same disease taking sugar pills. The question we are asking is whether people live longer or shorter with the new drug, not whether they live forever."

"I can just imagine how upset the Social Security computer people will be to hear your idea; it sounds like a lot of work for them."

"Well, that just makes them feel more important. They probably would somewhat resist the idea because it brings new users into their private world. They must have a lot of errors in a big system like that, and at the moment nobody knows it but them. If a lot of scientists started using the system, the errors would get a lot more publicity. Hey, Opol! Do you have to make so much noise with that saw?"

"How many posts are you doing these days?"

"Less than a hundred a year. We used to do at least three hundred. It's like that everywhere, nowadays. Doctors are afraid we'll make trouble for them."

"Baloney. It's an unreimbursed loser for the pathologists."

"Well, it's a loser, all right," replied the pathologist. "I'll bet it costs us two thousand dollars to do one autopsy. You can't charge anybody for it, and mostly no one comes to watch. If you think about it, it's nearly a quarter of a million dollars a year that has to be buried in the budget."

"And if you were doing three hundred a year, would you lose three-quarters of a million? Your phone is ringing."

"Of course not, you know better than that. It would cost the same quarter of a million. Would you answer the phone for us? Both Opol and I have gloves on."

The physician spectator picked up the phone. "It's an undertaker on the line. He wants to know if you have someone named O'Toole."

"I don't know," said the pathologist, "take a look in the icebox." The other doctor walked over to a large walk-in refrigerator, pulled hard on the noisy handle of the heavy door, and walked in.

"Where's the light?"

"The switch is outside on the wall."

"OK. Now how do I tell if O'Toole is here?"

"Look at the tag on the big toes."

"Oh, yes. He's here."

"Thanks. Just tell the undertaker, would you?"

27

What Should Be Done?

The reader has a right to know what I would propose to do about the problems described in this book. True, it seems a little unfair to link the adequacy of a proposed solution to the validity of a critical analysis; but that is something we all do in argumentation. It's a way of bringing out hidden motives. It's also a way of seeing whether a set of problems might be so insoluble that there is no "sense" in complaining about them.

My first proposal is that we undertake a movement back to self-insurance for ordinary health expenses. I do not propose that first-dollar coverage should be outlawed or even held up to ridicule. It is only necessary that public awareness be stimulated to understand the costliness of pre-paying small items through insurance and of the upward pressure it puts on medical prices. If there is sufficient public awareness of the advantages of self-insurance, there will then be enough public resistance to national schemes of "universal comprehensive" benefits which would make self-insurance impossible. One more qualifier: Truly poor people are outside the marketplace, and some degree of special treatment of ordinary medical expenses must be made in their behalf.

A second proposal is that we strongly encourage the use of high deductible insurance as a means of paying for extraordinary medical expenses. I'm a little scared of the potential inflationary consequences of developing a federal system of health catastrophe insurance, and would much prefer to see a competitive system of private health insurance companies provide the coverage. I do hope private companies will see the public duty to respond to this need. In many ways, it could be said that the failure of the commercial health insurance industry to respond to the needs of the 1930's was the start of our long romance with nonmarket health care systems. As we saw in the chapter on the subject, I believe the most feasible incremental way of achieving self-insurance for ordinary health costs is to start at the high end with health catastrophe protection and allow the public to decide how much of the amount at the bottom end it would like to self-insure. If the industry fails to provide such a vehicle, the public will be afraid to drop first-dollar coverage. Once it becomes more easily possible to buy cheap catastrophe protection, the whole matter of supplemental insurance will suddenly become legitimized. In our present upside-down system, the purchase of gap-filling insurance defeats the usage restraints of co-insurance and deductibles. But if the top layer were covered first, the premium price of each layer downward would allow people to decide how much they wanted to pay for how much risk protection. In the example in the earlier chapter, there was one layer where you would have to pay $350 a year extra premium to protect yourself against a potential loss of $500. You would have to be pretty timid to pay that price for protection, but it would be your money, and your choice. In my opinion, most people buy gap-filling supplemental coverage because they don't know how high their bills might go, and want to get as much covered as they can. If they knew exactly how high the bill could go and no higher, they might be less hysterical and could afford to be more shrewd with their money. This whole matter will take lots of public education. I wrote this book to extend the reach of my voice on the subject, but there's nothing like an army of commission-reimbursed insurance salesmen to spread the word.

My next proposal is that we adopt a national goal of gradually removing the tax subsidy for health insurance. It seems a good idea to me to encourage self-insurance by removing the tax-subsidy from the anti-social first-dollar lower end. If I were a Congressman, I would try to get agreement through extending the subsidy to all taxpayers on the high end along with simultaneously removing it from the low end. That way, the people who stood to have the present inequity removed would help shout down those who were resisting the loss of the special privilege. The tax-subsidy could be made uniform at a certain dollar amount and then frozen at that level. In time, inflation would shrink the value of the subsidy to a trivial level. Does that sound cynical? In any event, one way or another, this tax incentive to overextend health insurance benefits should be phased out.

Next, we must stop the system of cost reimbursement to hospitals. Paying their prices instead of their costs would result in some short-run cost increase before the long-run economies began to appear. Some of this could be offset by the increased tax revenues from eliminating tax-subsidy to health insurance. I would also propose that the offer to pay prices rather than costs should only be extended to hospitals who expose their profit to federal corporation tax. And this tax recapture ought to soften the blow to the federal treasury still further.

But it will still probably cost something at first, and there is no sense in saying it won't. Wouldn't it be wonderful if we could get more people (in and out of Congress) to understand that you must spend money to save money? If we saw that more clearly on a national level, we might start to give the Japanese a better run for it in international trade.

Next, other incentives must be devised to persuade more non-profit hospitals to spin off their revenue centers into tax-paying subsidiaries. The permissable level of profitability should be examined for its incentives to hospitals to shift their corporate form. Conditional relaxation of the rules about simultaneous borrowing and lending should be used as a lever.

In order to stimulate some cost-consciousness among consumers, there should be a voluntary effort to have employees pay their own premiums, and patients pay their own bills, even though employers might be providing the money for the premium, and insurance might be reimbursing the cost of the medical bill. It shouldn't be too difficult to adjust the IRS regulations to permit the premium transfer without affecting the tax-shelter (assuming we can't get rid of the tax-shelter). And it shouldn't be too difficult for hospitals to wait for their payments until the reimbursement occurs, since they are now waiting anyway. The assignment of benefits is a pernicious short-cut, whose cost-saving feature is mostly illusory.

Next, we must do something about the staggering tax-subsidy we extend to hospital municipal revenue bonds. Not only does this subsidize construction which the HSAs are fruitlessly created to restrain, but it is subversive to the national effort to control inflation through raising general interest rates. Under the cost-reimbursement system, hospitals have only a minor reason to be restrained by interest rates.

And finally, there should be a nation-wide meeting to get all hospitals to be born again on the subject of fully funded depreciation. If you don't know what that means after all of those earlier chapters, don't worry about it. Just echo the slogan. Take it from me, it would help a lot. It is the only mechanism I can see to prevent a nationwide, absolute moratorium on all new hospital construction, which would be just as hideous a situation as the present rush to over-enhance.

Let's just list these eight proposals:

- Self-insurance for ordinary expenses (except for the indigent).
- High-deductible, non-nationalized coverage for extraordinary expenses.
- Gradual elimination of health insurance income tax subsidy.
- Elimination of cost reimbursement, whether retrospective or prospective.
- Encouragement of hospitals to develop taxable subsidiaries.
- Curtailment of the assignment of benefits, and encouragement of employee payment of health insurance premiums.
- Reform of the tax-free municipal bond system for hospital construction projects.
- Full funding of depreciation.

When you look over that list, you see that there are a lot of big words from insurance jargon in those proposals. Let's try again in simpler language:

- Pay cash for medical expenses if you possibly can.
- Only buy health insurance protection against bills that would really wipe you out.
- Close the income-tax loophole on health insurance fringe benefits.
- Make everybody pay the same amount for the same hospital service, but include a profit margin.
- Let hospitals earn a profit, but make them pay taxes.
- Pay your own insurance premium, and pay your own medical bills, even though you are repaid for them.
- Limit the use of tax-exempt bond funding to prospectuses

which have been approved by the SEC, and to situations when there is a demonstrated waiting list for the proposed facility.
- Make hospitals establish a sinking fund for building replacement, and keep it paid up at all times.

Is that all we should do? Of course not. We need to continue to fund and assist scientific research, so that the one-time cost of eliminating a disease can replace the endless process of curing it, while the cost of curing other diseases can replace the staggering cost of having them. It is pleasing to see Congress give a billion dollars this year to my old employer, the National Cancer Institute. That's enough for cancer, but you could give the whole $5 billion we spent on hospital construction last year to other research, as far as I am concerned.

We need to find ways of transforming the enormous domestic health system into an export industry, with consequent benefit to our international balance of payments.

We need to computerize and rationalize the archaic system of scientific information storage and retrieval, which is in turn linked to the $3.6 billion industry known as Continuing Medical Education.

We need to be able to determine the ultimate longevity of people treated, in some defined manner, and this needs to be compared with the retrospective cost and characteristics of the provider. The Social Security System, compelled to stop payments at the death of a client, makes a simple tool for accomplishing this elementary task of determining in retrospect what good it all was, and how much extra longevity we got for how much cost.

We need to force a confrontation between the concept of quackery as freedom of trade, on the one hand, and simultaneous insistence on impossible standards of malpractice for scientific practitioners, on the other. You cannot have it both ways; either quackery is to be eliminated or malpractice is to be ignored.

We need to find ways of diverting the coming glut of physicians into a reassertion of the role of physicians in setting health policy and administering hospitals. The principal reason so few hospitals are now run by physicians is that physicians are in too short supply.

We need lots of other things. Perhaps we need another book on the subject, but I am already reminded of the prayer attributed to Job: "Would that mine enemy should write a book."